JUNE 1995

# GLOSSARY OF HIV/AIDS-RELATED TERMS

HIV/AIDS TREATMENT INFORMATION SERVICE
1-800-HIV-0440

# INTRODUCTION

The Glossary of HIV-Related Terms was compiled to define words that are commonly used to describe the HIV virus, its pathogenesis, its associated treatments, and the medical management of related conditions.

The glossary contains many up-to-date terms associated with this disease. Not every technical term has been included because of the enormity of such an undertaking. This glossary will help readers define the most common technical terms associated with HIV.

The six PHS agencies that co-sponsor the HIV/AIDS Treatment Information Service (ATIS) were instrumental in supporting this effort. ATIS, the newest component of the Centers for Disease Control and Prevention National AIDS Clearinghouse, is a free telephone reference service for health care providers and people with HIV infection. It provides the latest information about federally approved treatment guidelines. With the number of approved treatment guidelines increasing each year, it is essential for care providers and people living with HIV/AIDS to have one place to call for current treatment information.

The number to call for the HIV/AIDS Treatment Information Service is:

800–448–0440 (Voice)
800–243–7012 (Deaf Access/TDD)
301–738–6616 (Fax)

We hope that you find the Glossary of HIV-Related Terms helpful. If you would like additional information about ATIS and/or the other resources at the CDC National AIDS Clearinghouse, please call the Clearinghouse at:

800–458–5231 (Voice)
800–243–7012 (Deaf Access/TDD)
301–738–6616 (Fax)

The Clearinghouse also offers the following additional HIV/AIDS information Services:

## AIDS CLINICAL TRIALS INFORMATION SERVICE

AIDS Clinical Trials Information Service (ACTIS) provides up-to-date information on clinical trials that evaluate experimental drugs and other therapies for adults and children at all stages of HIV infection.

800–874–2572 (Voice)
800–243–7012 (Deaf Access/TDD)
301–738–6616 (Fax)

## BUSINESS AND LABOR RESOURCE SERVICE

Business and Labor Resource Service (BLRS) is a centralized information and referral service that links the business and labor communities with resources for developing HIV/AIDS in the workplace programs.

800–458–5231 (Voice)
800–243–7012 (Deaf Access/TDD)
301–738–6616 (Fax)

All of the HIV/AIDS reference services operate Monday through Friday from 9:00a.m. to 7:00p.m., E.S.T. All calls are completely confidential.

The PHS agencies who sponsor the HIV/AIDS Treatment Information Service and this glossary are:

Agency for Health Care Policy and Research
Centers for Disease Control and Prevention
Health Resources and Services Administration
Indian Health Service
National Institutes of Health
Office of HIV/AIDS Policy
Substance Abuse and Mental Health Services Administration

# HIV/AIDS GLOSSARY

# A

## ACQUIRED IMMUNODEFICIENCY SYNDROME (AIDS):

The most severe manifestation of infection with the human immunodeficiency virus (HIV). The Centers for Disease Control and Prevention list numerous opportunistic infections and neoplasms (cancers) which, in the presence of HIV infection, constitute an AIDS diagnosis. In addition, a CD4+ T-cell count below $200/mm^3$ in the presence of HIV infection constitutes an AIDS diagnosis. The period between infection with HIV and the onset of AIDS averages 10 years in the United States. People with AIDS often suffer infections of the lungs, brain, eyes and other organs, and frequently suffer debilitating weight loss, diarrhea and a type of cancer called Kaposi's sarcoma. Even with treatment, most people with AIDS die within two years of developing infections or cancers that take advantage of their weakened immune systems. See also CD4 (T4) or CD4+ Cells; Diarrhea; HIV Disease; Kaposi's Sarcoma; Opportunistic Infection; Wasting Syndrome.

## ACROMEGALY:

A chronic disease caused by hypersecretion of the pituitary growth hormones. It is characterized by enlargement of many parts of the skeleton, especially the nose, ears, jaws, fingers and toes. See also Pituitary Gland.

## ACTG:

See AIDS Clinical Trials Group.

## ACUTE INFECTION:

An infection causing disease with a sudden onset, severity and (often) short course. As related to HIV infection: Once the virus enters the body, HIV infects a large number of CD4+ T cells and replicates rapidly. During this acute or primary phase of infection, the blood contains many viral particles that spread throughout the body, seeding themselves in various organs, particularly the lymphoid tissues. See also Acute Retroviral Syndrome; CD4 (T4) or CD4+ Cells; Infection; Lymphoid Organs.

**ACUTE RETROVIRAL SYNDROME:**
The acute or primary HIV infection often passes unrecognized, but may be present as a mononucleosis-like syndrome within three months of the infection. The diagnosis is made by demonstrating HIV antibody seroconversion. See also Seroconversion.

**ACYCLOVIR:**
(Acycloguanosine). A nucleoside analog antiviral drug used to treat the symptoms of the genital form of herpes simplex virus infection. See also Herpes Simplex Virus; Nucleoside Analog.

**ADENOPATHY:**
Any disease involving or causing enlargement of glandular tissues, especially one involving the lymph nodes.

**ADJUVANT:**
An ingredient—as in a prescription or solution—that facilitates or modifies the action of the principal ingredient. May be used in HIV therapies or for HIV vaccines.

**ADMINISTRATION:**
(Route of Administration). A term used to refer to how a drug or therapy is introduced into the body. *Systemic administration* means that the drug goes throughout the body (usually carried in the bloodstream), and includes oral administration (by mouth) and intravenous administration (injection into the vein). *Local administration* means that the drug is applied or introduced into the specific area affected by the disease, such as application directly onto the affected skin surface (topical administration). The effects of most therapies depend upon the ability of the drug to reach the affected area, thus the route of adminis-

tration and consequent distribution of a drug in the body is an important determinant of its effectiveness.

### ADVERSE EVENT:
In a clinical trial, an unwanted effect detected in participants. The term is used whether or not the effect can be attributed to the intervention under study.

### ADVERSE REACTION:
See Side Effects.

### AEROSOLIZED:
A form of administration in which a drug, such as pentamidine, is turned into a fine spray or mist by a nebulizer and inhaled. See also Pentamidine.

### AETC:
See AIDS Education and Training Centers.

### AFFECTED COMMUNITY:
This includes HIV-positive people, persons living with AIDS and other individuals, including their families, friends and advocates, directly impacted by HIV infection and its physical, psychological and sociological ramifications.

### AGAMMAGLOBULINEMIA:
A nearly total absence of immunoglobulins. See also Antibodies.

### AGENCY FOR HEALTH CARE POLICY AND RESEARCH (AHCPR):
An agency of the Public Health Service that supports activities to enhance health care services and improve access to them.

### AHCPR:
See Agency for Health Care Policy and Research.

## AIDS:
See Acquired Immunodeficiency Syndrome.

## AIDS BIBLIOGRAPHY:
The National Library of Medicine publishes the monthly *AIDS Bibliography*, which includes all citations from the AIDSLINE database. The *AIDS Bibliography* is available from the Superintendent of Documents (Phone: 202–783–3238). See also AIDSLINE.

## AIDS CLINICAL TRIALS GROUP (ACTG):
The ACTG is composed of a number of US medical centers that evaluate treatment for HIV and HIV-associated infections. ACTG studies are sponsored by the National Institute of Allergy and Infectious Diseases.

## AIDS DEMENTIA COMPLEX:
About half the people infected with HIV, the virus that causes AIDS, develop infections or other problems involving the brain or spinal cord. These neurological complications may include inflammation of the brain (encephalitis), or of the membrane surrounding the brain (meningitis), infections of the brain, brain or spinal cord tumors, nerve damage, difficulties in thinking and behavioral changes (i.e., AIDS dementia complex) and stroke.

## AIDSDRUGS:
An online database service administered by the National Library of Medicine, with references to drugs undergoing testing against AIDS, AIDS-related complex and related opportunistic infections.

## AIDS EDUCATION AND TRAINING CENTERS (AETC):
The Health Resources and Services Administration supports a network of 15 regional centers that serve as resources for educating health professionals in prevention, diagnosis and care of HIV-infected patients. The centers train primary caregivers to incorporate HIV prevention strategies into their clinical priorities, along with diagnosis, counseling and care of HIV-infected persons and their families.

## AIDS KNOWLEDGE BASE:

Full-text electronic database on AIDS, available in print as well as electronic form, produced and maintained by physicians and other health care professionals. The database is edited by P.T. Cohen (San Francisco General Hospital), Merle Sande, and Paul Volberding.

## AIDSLINE:

An online database service administered by the National Library of Medicine, with citations and abstracts covering the published scientific and medical literature on AIDS and related topics.

## AIDS-RELATED CANCERS:

Several cancers are more common or more aggressive in people infected with HIV, the virus that causes AIDS. These malignancies include certain types of immune system cancers known as lymphomas, Kaposi's sarcoma and anogenital cancers primarily affecting the cervix and the anus. HIV, or the immune suppression it induces, appears to play a role in the development of these cancers. See also Cervical Cancer; Kaposi's Sarcoma; Lymphoma.

## AIDS-RELATED COMPLEX (ARC):

1. A term, not officially defined or recognized by the Centers for Disease Control and Prevention, that has been used to describe a variety of symptoms and signs found in some persons infected with HIV. These may include recurrent fevers, unexplained weight loss, swollen lymph nodes, and/or fungus infection of the mouth and throat. Also commonly described as symptomatic HIV infection. 2. Symptoms that appear to be related to infection by the HIV virus. They include an unexplained, chronic deficiency of white blood cells (leukopenia) or a poorly functioning lymphatic system with swelling of the lymph nodes (lymphadenopathy) lasting for more than three months without the opportunistic infections required for a diagnosis of AIDS. See also Wasting Syndrome.

**AIDS RESEARCH ADVISORY COMMITTEE:**
Board that advises and makes recommendations to the Director, National Institute of Allergy and Infectious Diseases, on all aspects of HIV-related research, vaccine development, pathogenesis and epidemiology.

**AIDS SERVICE ORGANIZATION (ASO):**
A health association, support agency or other service active in the prevention and treatment of AIDS.

**AIDSTRIALS:**
An online database service administered by the National Library of Medicine, with information about clinical trials of agents under evaluation against HIV infection, AIDS and related opportunistic infections.

**AIDS WASTING SYNDROME:**
See Wasting Syndrome.

**ALKALINE PHOSPHATASE:**
An enzyme that is normally present in certain cells within the liver, bone, kidney, intestine and placenta. When the cells are destroyed in those tissues, more of the enzyme leaks into the blood, and levels rise in proportion to the severity of the condition. Measurement of this enzyme is used as an indication of the health of the liver.

**ALOPECIA:**
The loss of hair that frequently occurs in patients undergoing chemotherapy for cancer or suffering from other diseases, such as AIDS, where cell-killing, or cytotoxic, drugs are used.

**ALTERNATIVE THERAPY:**
In Western countries, alternative therapy refers to any type of medicine that supplements or is used in lieu of biomedicine (i.e., conventional medicine) or allopathic medicine. In other parts of the world, where traditional medicine predominates, the term may refer to biomedicine itself.

**ALUM:**
Potassium aluminum sulfate or ammonium aluminum sulfate, used especially as an emetic (i.e., an agent that induces vomiting), an astringent (i.e., a substance that contracts tissues) and styptic (i.e., a substance that tends to check bleeding by contracting the tissues or blood vessels).

**ALVEOLAR:**
Pertaining to the alveoli sac, the site of gas exchange in the lungs.

**AMEBIASIS:**
An inflammation of the intestines caused by infestation with *Entameba histolytica* (a type of ameba) and characterized by frequent, loose stools flecked with blood and mucus.

**AMINO ACIDS:**
Any of a class of organic compounds having a carboxyl group (COOH) and an amino group ($NH^2$). Some 22 amino acids are commonly found in animals, and more than 100 less common forms are found in nature, chiefly in plants. When the carboxyl carbon atom of one amino acid binds to the nitrogen of another with the release of a water molecule, a linkage called a peptide bond is formed. Chains of amino acids, joined head-to-tail in this manner, are synthesized by living systems and are called polypeptides (up to about 50 amino acids) and proteins (over 50 amino acids). See also Peptide; Proteins.

**AMNIOCENTESIS:**
The surgical insertion of a hollow needle through the abdominal wall and into the uterus of a pregnant female to obtain amniotic fluid (i.e., the serous fluid in which the embryo is suspended) especially to examine the fetal chromosomes for an abnormality or for the determination of the sex of the embryo. See also Uterus.

**ANALOG:**
In chemistry, a compound with a structure similar to that of another compound, but differing from it in respect to certain components or

structural makeup; it may have a similar or opposite action metabolically.

**ANAMNESTIC RESPONSE:**
The heightened immunologic reaction elicited by a second or subsequent exposure to a particular pathogenic microorganism or antigen. See also Antigen.

**ANAPHYLACTIC SHOCK:**
A life-threatening allergic reaction characterized by a swelling of body tissues (including the throat) and a sudden decline in blood pressure.

**ANEMIA:**
A lower than normal number of red blood cells.

**ANERGY:**
1. The loss or weakening of the body's immunity to an irritating agent, or antigen. The strength of the body's immune response is often quantitatively measured by means of a skin test where a solution containing an antigen known to cause a response, such as mumps or candida, is injected immediately under the skin. The lack of a reaction to these common antigens indicates anergy. See also Antigen. 2. Researchers in cell culture have shown that CD4+ T cells can be turned off by a signal from HIV that leaves them unable to respond to further immune system stimulation. This inactivated state is known as anergy. See also CD4 (T4) or CD4+ Cells.

**ANTIBIOTIC:**
An antimicrobial agent, derived from cultures of a microorganism or produced semisynthetically, used to treat infections.

**ANTIBODIES:**
Molecules in the blood or secretory fluids that tag, destroy or neutralize bacteria, viruses or other harmful toxins. They are members of a class of proteins known as immunoglobulins, which are produced and secreted

by B lymphocytes in response to stimulation by antigens. An antibody is specific to an antigen. See also Antigen; Lymphocyte.

### ANTIBODY-DEPENDENT CELL-MEDIATED CYTOTOXICITY (ADCC):

An immune response in which antibodies bind to target cells, identifying them for attack by the immune system. See also Antibodies.

### ANTIFOLATE:

An agent that inhibits intracellular (i.e., inside cells) production of folinic acid. See also Folinic Acid.

### ANTIGEN:

A substance that, when introduced into the body, is capable of inducing the production of a specific antibody. See also Antibodies.

### ANTIIDIOTYPE:

An antibody that recognizes and binds to another antibody (idiotype).

### ANTINEOPLASTIC:

Inhibiting or preventing the proliferation of tumor cells.

### ANTIRETROVIRAL AGENTS:

Substances used against retroviruses such as HIV. See also Retrovirus.

### ANTITOXINS:

Antibodies that recognize and inactivate toxins produced by certain bacteria, plants or animals. See also Antibodies.

### ANTIVIRAL:

A substance or process that destroys a virus or suppresses its replication.

**APOPTOSIS:**
Cellular suicide, also known as programmed cell death. HIV may induce apoptosis in both infected and uninfected immune system cells. Uninfected cells may also undergo apoptosis. Normally when CD4+ T cells mature in the thymus gland, a small proportion of these cells are unable to distinguish self from nonself. Because these cells would otherwise attack the body's own tissues, they receive a biochemical signal from other cells that results in apoptosis. See also CD4 (T4) or CD4+ Cells; Thymus.

**ARC:**
See AIDS-Related Complex.

**ARM:**
A group of participants in a clinical trial, all of whom receive the same treatment or placebo. See also Placebo.

**ARTHRALGIA:**
A pain in a joint.

**ASO:**
See AIDS Service Organization.

**ASPERGILLOSIS:**
A fungal infection (resulting from the fungus *Aspergillus*) of the lungs that can spread through the blood to other organs. Symptoms include fever, chills, difficulty in breathing and coughing up blood. If the infection reaches the brain, it may cause dementia. See also Dementia.

**ASSEMBLY AND BUDDING:**
Names for a portion of the processes by which new HIV virus is formed in infected host cells. Viral core proteins, enzymes and RNA (ribonucleic acid) gather just inside the cell's membrane, while the viral envelope proteins aggregate within the membrane. An immature viral particle is formed and then pinches off from the cell, acquiring an

envelope and the cellular and HIV proteins from the cell membrane. The immature viral particle then undergoes processing by an HIV enzyme called protease to become an infectious virus. See also Enzyme; Ribonucleic Acid.

### ASYMPTOMATIC:
Without symptoms. Usually used in AIDS literature to describe a person who has a positive reaction to one of several tests for HIV antibodies, but who shows no clinical symptoms of the disease.

### ATTENUATED:
Weakened or decreased. For example, an attenuated virus can no longer produce disease, but might be used to produce a vaccine.

### AUTOANTIBODY:
1. An antibody that is active against some of the tissues of the organism that produced it. 2. An antibody directed against the body's own tissue. See also Antibodies.

### AUTOIMMUNIZATION:
The induction in an individual of an immune response to its own cells (tissue). See also Immune Response.

### AUTOINOCULABLE:
Susceptible of being inoculated with microorganisms from one's own body.

### AUTOLOGOUS:
Pertaining to the same organism or one of its parts; originating within an organism itself.

### AZT:
Azidothymidine (also called zidovudine or ZDV; the Burroughs-Wellcome trade name is Retrovir). One of the first drugs used against HIV infection, AZT is a nucleoside analog that suppresses replication of HIV. See also Nucleoside Analog.

# B

**BACTERICIDAL:**
Capable of killing bacteria.

**BACTERIOSTATIC:**
Capable of inhibiting reproduction of bacteria.

**BACTERIUM:**
A microscopic organism composed of a single cell. Many bacteria can cause disease in humans.

**BACULOVIRUS:**
A virus of insects used in the production of some HIV vaccines. See also Vaccine.

**BASELINE:**
1. Information gathered at the beginning of a study from which variations found in the study are measured. 2. A known value or quantity with which an unknown is compared when measured or assessed.

**BASOPHIL:**
A type of white blood cell, also called a granular leukocyte, filled with granules of toxic chemicals that can digest microorganisms. Basophils, as well as other types of white blood cells, are responsible for the symptoms of allergy. The granules stain blue when exposed to a basic dye for microscopic examination.

**B CELL LYMPHOMA:**
See Lymphoma.

**B CELLS:**
See B Lymphocytes.

**BILIRUBIN:**
1. A bile pigment whose measurement can be used as an indication of the health of the liver. 2. A substance released from old or damaged red blood cells. Small amounts of bilirubin normally enter the bloodstream and circulate until they reach the liver and then into the bowel, where bilirubin is further broken down and excreted. The normal value is 0.1 to 1.5 milligrams per liter of blood.

**BINDING ANTIBODY:**
As related to HIV infection: An antibody that attaches to some part of the HIV virus. Binding antibodies may or may not adversely affect the virus.

**BIOLOGICAL RESPONSE MODIFIERS (BRMS):**
Substances, either natural or synthesized, that boost, direct or restore normal immune defenses. BRMs include interferons, interleukins, thymus hormones and monoclonal antibodies. See also Interferon; Interleukin-2; Monoclonal Antibody; Thymus.

**BIOPSY:**
The surgical removal of a piece of tissue from a living subject for microscopic examination to make a diagnosis (for example, to determine whether abnormal cells such as cancer cells are present).

**BIOTECHNOLOGY:**
1. The use of living organisms or their products to make or modify a substance. These include recombinant DNA techniques (also referred to as genetic engineering) and hybridoma technology. 2. The industrial application of the results of biological research, particularly in fields such as recombinant DNA or gene splicing, which permits the production of synthetic hormones or enzymes by combining genetic material from different species.

## BLINDED STUDY:

A clinical trial in which participants are unaware as to whether or not they are in the experimental or control arm of the study.

## BLOOD BRAIN BARRIER:

The barrier between brain blood vessels and brain tissues whose effect is to restrict what may pass from the blood into the brain.

## B LYMPHOCYTES (B CELLS):

One of the two major classes of lymphocytes. During infections, these cells are transformed into plasma cells that produce large quantities of antibody directed at specific pathogens. This transformation occurs through interactions with various types of T cells and other components of the immune system. In persons with AIDS, the functional ability of both the B and the T lymphocytes is damaged, with the T lymphocytes being the principal site of infection by the HIV virus. See also Lymphocyte; T Cells.

## BODY FLUIDS:

Any fluid in the human body, such as blood, urine, saliva, sputum (spit), tears, semen, mother's milk or vaginal secretions. Only blood, semen, mother's milk and vaginal secretions have been linked directly to the transmission of the HIV virus.

## BONE MARROW:

Soft tissue located in the cavities of the bones where blood cells such as erythrocytes, leukocytes and platelets are formed. See also Erythrocytes; Leukocytes; Platelets.

## BOOSTER:

A second or later dose of a vaccine given to increase the immune response to the original dose. See also Vaccine.

## BRANCHED DNA ASSAY:

A sensitive, rapid test that can be used to monitor the amount of HIV in a patient's bloodstream (i.e., the viral burden). See also Viral Burden.

## BREAKTHROUGH INFECTION:

An infection, caused by the infectious agent the vaccine is designed to protect against, that occurs during the course of a vaccine trial. These infections may be caused by exposure to the infectious agent before the vaccine has taken effect, or before all doses of the vaccine have been given. Breakthrough infections also occur in trial participants receiving placebos.

## BRONCHOSCOPY:

Visual examination of the bronchial passages of the lungs through a tube of an endoscope inserted into the upper lungs or extraction of material from the lungs by means of a bronchoscope. See also Endoscopy.

## BUDDING:

See Assembly and Budding.

## BURKITT'S LYMPHOMA:

A lymphatic cancer that involves not only the lymphatic and the associated reticuloendothelial system, but also other body tissues. This disease, which is most common in Central Africa, is thought to be possibly caused by the Epstein-Barr virus. Also called African lymphoma, Burkitt's tumor. See also Epstein-Barr Virus; Lymph; Reticuloendothelial Cells.

# C

## CACHEXIA:
General ill health and malnutrition, marked by weakness and emaciation, usually associated with serious disease. See also Wasting Syndrome.

## CANDIDA:
Yeast-like fungi commonly found in the normal flora of the mouth, skin, intestinal tract and vagina, but can become clinically infectious in immune compromised people. See also Fungus.

## CANDIDIASIS:
An infection with a fungus of the Candida family, generally *Candida albicans*; it most commonly involves the skin (dermatocandidiasis), oral mucosa (thrush), respiratory tract (bronchocandidiasis) and vagina (vaginitis). Candidiasis of the esophagus, trachea, bronchi or lungs is an indicator disease for AIDS. See also Fungus; Thrush.

## CARCINOGEN:
Any cancer-producing substance.

## CATHETER:
A tubular medical device for insertion into canals, vessels, passageways or body cavities, usually to permit injection (e.g., through an intravenous catheter into a vein) or withdrawal of fluids, or to keep a passage open.

## CBCT:
See Community-Based Clinical Trial.

## CBO:
See Community-Based Organization.

## CDC:

See Centers for Disease Control and Prevention.

## CD8 (T8) CELLS:

A protein embedded in the cell surface of suppressor T lymphocytes. Also called cytotoxic T cells. See also CD Nomenclature; CD4 (T4) or CD4+ Cells; T Cells.

## CD4 (T4) OR CD4 CELLS:

1. White blood cells killed or disabled during HIV infection. These cells normally orchestrate the immune response, signaling other cells in the immune system to perform their special functions. Also known as T helper cells. 2. HIV's preferred targets are cells that have a docking molecule called cluster designation 4 (CD4) on their surfaces. Cells with this molecule are known as CD4-positive (or CD4+) cells. Destruction of CD4+ lymphocytes is the major cause of the immunodeficiency observed in AIDS, and decreasing CD4+ lymphocyte levels appear to be the best indicator of morbidity in these patients. Although CD4 counts fall, the total T-cell level remains fairly constant through the course of HIV disease, due to a concomitant increase in the CD8+ cells. The ratio of CD4+ to CD8+ cells is therefore an important measure of disease progression. See also CD Nomenclature; CD8 (T8) Cells; Immunodeficiency.

## CDC NATIONAL AIDS CLEARINGHOUSE:

The CDC's comprehensive reference, referral and publication distribution service for HIV and AIDS information. The Clearinghouse works in partnership with national, regional, state and local organizations that develop and deliver HIV prevention programs and services.

## CD NOMENCLATURE:

This nomenclature was developed to standardize and compare monoclonal antibodies from different sources. Antibodies with similar reactivity patterns are assigned to CD groups representing "clusters of differentiation." T lymphocytes are CD3+ and can be separated into the

CD4+ T helper cells and the CD8+ cytotoxic/suppressor cells. Although CD4+ cells are predominantly T lymphocytes, some monocytes are also CD4+.

**CELL LINES:**
Specific cell types artificially maintained in the laboratory (i.e., in vitro) for scientific purposes.

**CELL-MEDIATED IMMUNITY (CMI):**
The branch of the immune system in which the reaction to foreign material is performed by specific defense cells (i.e., killer cells, macrophage and other white blood cells) rather than antibodies.

**CELLULAR IMMUNITY:**
See Cell-Mediated Immunity.

**CENTERS FOR DISEASE CONTROL AND PREVENTION (CDC):**
A Public Health Service agency responsible (among others) for assessing the status and characteristics of the AIDS epidemic and the prevalence of HIV infections. CDC supports the design, implementation and evaluation of prevention activities, and maintains various HIV/AIDS information services, such as the CDC National AIDS Clearinghouse.

**CENTRAL NERVOUS SYSTEM (CNS):**
Composed of the brain, spinal cord and its coverings (meninges).

**CENTRAL NERVOUS SYSTEM (CNS) DAMAGE:**
(By HIV infection). Although monocytes and macrophages can be infected by HIV, they appear to be relatively resistant to killing. However, these cells travel throughout the body and carry HIV to various organs, especially the lungs and the brain. People infected with HIV often experience abnormalities in the central nervous system. Investigators have hypothesized that an accumulation of HIV in brain and nerve cells or the inappropriate release of cytokines or toxic byproducts by

these cells may be to blame for the neurological manifestations of HIV disease. See also Cytokines; Macrophage; Monocyte.

**CEREBRAL:**
Pertaining to the cerebrum, the main portion of the brain.

**CERVICAL CANCER:**
A neoplasm of the uterine cervix that can be detected in the early curable stage by the Papanicolaou (Pap) test. See also Cervical Dysplasia; Cervix; Pap Smear.

**CERVICAL DYSPLASIA:**
A precursor lesion for cervical cancer. Studies indicate an increase in prevalence of cervical dysplasia among HIV-infected women. Additional studies have documented that a higher prevalence is associated with greater immunosuppression. HIV infection also may adversely affect the clinical course and treatment of cervical dysplasia and cancer. See also Dysplasia.

**CERVICAL INTRAEPITHELIAL NEOPLASIA (CIN1, CIN2, CIN3):**
Dysplasia of the cervix epithelium, often pre-malignant (i.e., cancerous), characterized by various degrees of hyperplasia, abnormal keratinization (forming horny epidermal tissue) and condylomata. Considerable evidence implicates human papilloma virus (HPV) in the development of CIN. Immunosuppression may also play an important role in facilitating infection or persistence of HPV in the genital tract and progression of HPV-induced neoplasia. See also Cervix; Condyloma; Dysplasia; Epithelium; Hyperplasia; Neoplasm.

**CERVIX:**
The part of the uterus that protrudes into the cavity of the vagina. See also Uterus.

## CHALLENGE:
In vaccine experiments, the exposure of an immunized animal to the infectious agent.

## CHEMOTHERAPY:
The treatment, mostly of cancer, by the use of a series of cytotoxic drugs that attack cancerous cells. This treatment commonly has adverse side effects that may include the temporary loss of the body's natural immunity to infections, loss of hair, digestive upset and a general feeling of illness. Although unpleasant, the adverse effects of treatment are tolerated considering the life-threatening nature of the cancers usually treated by chemotherapy. See also Cytotoxic.

## CHRONIC IDIOPATHIC DEMYELINATING POLYNEUROPATHY (CIPD):
Chronic, spontaneous loss or destruction of myelin. Myelin is a soft, white, somewhat fatty material that forms a thick sheath around the protoplasmic core of myelinated nerve fiber.

## CIPD:
See Chronic Idiopathic Demyelinating Polyneuropathy.

## CIRCULATING IMMUNE COMPLEXES:
See Immune Complex.

## CLADE:
A group of related HIV variants, classified according to degree of genetic similarity. HIV variants are currently grouped into clades A, B, C, D, E, F and O.

## CLINICAL:
Pertaining to or founded on observation and treatment of patients, as distinguished from theoretical or basic science.

## CLINICAL ALERT:

A mechanism, adopted by the National Institutes of Health in conjunction with the editors of several biomedical journals, for urgent cases in which timely and broad dissemination of results of clinical trials could prevent morbidity (sickness) and mortality (death). The Clinical Alert does not become a barrier to subsequent publication of the full research paper. Clinical Alerts are widely distributed electronically through the National Library of Medicine and through standard mailings.

## CLINICAL LATENCY:

The state or period of an infectious agent, such as a virus or bacterium, living or developing in a host without producing clinical symptoms. As related to HIV infection: Although infected individuals usually exhibit a period of clinical latency with little evidence of disease, the virus is never truly latent. Even early in the disease, HIV is active within lymphoid organs where large amounts of virus become trapped in the FDC network. Surrounding germinal centers are areas rich in CD4+ T cells. These cells increasingly become infected and viral particles accumulate both in infected cells and as free virus. See also CD4 (T4) or CD4+ Cells; Lymphoid Organs.

## CLINICAL PRACTICE GUIDELINES:

Standards for physicians to adhere to in prescribing care for a given condition or illness.

## CLINICAL TRIAL:

A carefully designed and executed investigation of the effects of a drug (or vaccine) administered to human subjects. The goal is to define the clinical efficacy and pharmacological effects (toxicity, side effects, incompatibilities or interactions) of the drug. The US government, through the Food and Drug Administration, requires strict testing of all new drugs and vaccines prior to their approval for use as therapeutic agents.

## CLONE:

1. A group of genetically identical cells or organisms descended from a common ancestor. To produce such genetically identical copies. 2. A genetically identical replication of a living cell that is valuable for the investigation and reproduction of test cultures.

## CMV:

See Cytomegalovirus.

## CNS:

See Central Nervous System.

## COCCIDIOIDOMYCOSIS:

An infectious fungal disease caused by the inhalation of spores of *Coccidioides immitis,* which is carried on windblown dust particles. The disease is endemic in hot dry regions of the Southwestern US and Central and South America, and is an opportunistic disease associated with AIDS. Also called desert fever, San Joaquin fever, valleyfever. See also Fungus; Opportunistic Infection.

## COFACTORS:

1. Substances, microorganisms or characteristics of individuals that may influence the progression of a disease or the likelihood of becoming ill. 2. A substance, such as a metallic ion or coenzyme, that must be associated with an enzyme for the enzyme to function. 3. A situation or activity that may increase a person's susceptibility to AIDS. Examples of such cofactors are other infections, drugs and alcohol use, poor nutrition, genetic factors and stress.

## COHORT:

In epidemiology, a group of individuals with some characteristics in common.

## COLITIS:

Inflammation of the colon.

## COMMUNITY-BASED CLINICAL TRIAL (CBCT):

A clinical trial conducted primarily through primary-care physicians rather than academic research facilities.

## COMMUNITY-BASED ORGANIZATION (CBO):

A locally based service organization that provides social services at the community level.

## COMMUNITY PROGRAMS FOR CLINICAL RESEARCH ON AIDS (CPCRA):

An initiative of the National Institute of Allergy and Infectious Diseases (NIAID) to broaden the base of clinical investigations by involving community physicians in AIDS research and trials. NIAID started the CPCRA in 1989. It is one of four HIV clinical trials programs supported by NIAID. In 1992 the name of the program was officially changed to the Terry Beirn Community Programs for Clinical Research on AIDS. (See also Terry Beirn Community Programs for Clinical Research on AIDS).

## COMPASSIONATE USE:

A method of providing experimental drugs to very sick patients who have no other treatment options. Often, case-by-case approval must be obtained from the Food and Drug Administration for "compassionate use" of a drug.

## COMPLEMENT:

A group of proteins in normal blood serum and plasma which, in combination with antibodies, causes the destruction of antigens, particularly bacteria and foreign blood corpuscles. See also Antibodies; Antigen.

## COMPLEMENT CASCADE:

A precise sequence of events, usually triggered by an antigen-antibody complex, in which each component of the complement system is activated in turn. See also Antibodies; Antigen.

**CONCOMITANT DRUGS:**
Drugs that are taken together. Certain concomitant medications may have adverse interactions.

**CONCORDE STUDY:**
Joint French/British clinical trial of AZT in asymptomatic HIV-positive individuals. See also AZT.

**CONDYLOMA:**
(Condyloma acuminatum). A papilloma with a central core of connective tissue in a treelike structure covered with epithelium, usually occurring on the mucous membrane or skin of the external genitals or in the perianal (tissue surrounding the anus) region. Although the lesions are usually few in number, they may aggregate to form large cauliflower-like masses. Caused by the human papilloma virus (HPV), it is infectious and autoinoculable (i.e., capable of being transmitted by inoculation from one part of the body to another). Also called acuminate or venereal warts. See also Epithelium; Papilloma.

**CONTAGIOUS:**
Any infectious disease capable of being transmitted by casual contact from one person to another. Casual contact can be defined as normal day-to-day contact between people at home, school, work or in the community. A contagious infection (e.g., a common cold) can be communicable by casual contact; an infectious infection, on the other hand, is communicable by intimate contact such as sex. AIDS is infectious, not contagious.

**CONTRAINDICATION:**
A specific circumstance when the use of certain treatments could be harmful.

**CONTROL:**
A standard against which experimental observations may be evaluated. In clinical trials, one group of patients is given an experimental drug,

while another group (i.e., the control group) is given either a standard treatment for the disease or a placebo. See also Placebo.

### CORE PROTEIN:
As related to HIV: An integral protein of the HIV virus composed of three units, p24, p15 and p18.

### CORRELATES OF IMMUNITY/CORRELATES OF PROTECTION:
The immune responses that protect an individual from a certain disease. The precise identities of the correlates of immunity in HIV are unknown.

### CPCRA:
See Community Programs for Clinical Research on AIDS.

### CREATININE:
A protein found in muscles and blood, and excreted by the kidneys in the urine. The level of creatinine in the blood and urine provides a measure of kidney function.

### CRYPTOCOCCAL MENINGITIS:
A life-threatening infection of the membranes (meninges) that line the brain and the spinal cord. Cryptococcal disease is caused by a fungus (*Cryptococcus neoformans*). Most people have been exposed to this organism, which is found in soil contaminated by bird droppings, but it usually does not cause disease in healthy people. The majority of people with cryptococcal meningitis have immune systems that are damaged by disease, such as AIDS, or suppressed by drugs. The organism can infect almost all organs of the body, although it most commonly causes disease of the meninges, skin or lungs.

### CRYPTOCOCCOSIS:
An infectious disease seen in HIV-infected patients due to the fungus *Cryptococcus neoformans*, which is acquired via the respiratory tract. It can spread from the lungs to the brain, the central nervous system, the

skin, skeletal system and urinary tract. See also Cryptococcal Meningitis.

**CRYPTOSPORIDIOSIS:**
An opportunistic infection caused by the protozoan parasite *Cryptosporidium parvum.*

**CT:**
(Computed Tomography). Radiography (using X-rays) in which a three-dimensional image of a body structure is constructed by computer from a series of plane cross-sectional images made along an axis. Also referred to as CAT scan.

**CTL:**
See Cytotoxic T Lymphocyte.

**CUTANEOUS:**
Of, pertaining to or affecting the skin.

**CYTOKINES:**
1. Immune system proteins involved in the normal regulation of the immune response. They may also help to activate HIV-2. Proteins used for communication by cells of the immune system. Central to the normal regulation of the immune response.

**CYTOMEGALOVIRUS (CMV):**
A herpes virus that is a common cause of opportunistic diseases in people with AIDS and other people with immune suppression. While CMV can infect most organs of the body, people with AIDS are most susceptible to CMV retinitis (disease of the eye) and colitis (disease of the colon). See also Cytomegalovirus (CMV) Retinitis.

**CYTOMEGALOVIRUS (CMV) RETINITIS:**
Most adults in the US have been infected by cytomegalovirus, although the virus usually does not cause disease in healthy people. Because the

virus remains in the body for life, it can cause disease if the immune system becomes severely damaged by disease or suppressed by drugs. CMV retinitis is an eye disease common among people who are infected with HIV. Without treatment, people with CMV retinitis can lose their vision. CMV infection can affect both eyes and is the most common cause of blindness among people with AIDS.

**CYTOPENIA:**
Deficiency in the cellular elements of the blood.

**CYTOPLASM:**
All of the substance of a cell other than the nucleus.

**CYTOTOXIC:**
An agent or process that is toxic to cells (i.e., it causes suppression of function or cell death).

**CYTOTOXIC T LYMPHOCYTE (CTL):**
A lymphocyte that is able to kill foreign cells that have been marked for destruction by the cellular immune system. See also CD8 (T8) Cells; Lymphocyte.

# D

**DATABASE:**
An organized compilation of information, usually maintained in a computer system.

**DATA SAFETY AND MONITORING BOARD (DSMB):**
An independent committee, composed of community representatives and clinical research experts, that reviews data while a clinical trial is in progress to ensure that participants are not exposed to undue risk. A DSMB may recommend that a trial be stopped if there are safety concerns or if the trial objectives have been achieved.

**DATRI:**
See Division of AIDS Treatment Research Initiative.

**DDC:**
Dideoxycytidine (zalcitabine, HIVID), a nucleoside analog drug that inhibits the replication of HIV. See also Nucleoside Analog.

**DDI:**
Dideoxyinosine (didanosine, Videx), a nucleoside analog drug that inhibits the replication of HIV. See also Nucleoside Analog.

**DELETION:**
Elimination of a gene (i.e., from a chromosome) either in nature or in the laboratory. See also Gene.

**DEMENTIA:**
Chronic intellectual impairment (i.e., loss of mental capacity) with organic origins that affects a person's ability to function in a social or occupational setting. See also AIDS Dementia Complex.

## DEMYELINATION:

Destruction, removal or loss of the myelin sheath of a nerve or nerves. See also Myelin.

## DENDRITE:

Any of the usual branching protoplasmic processes that conduct impulses toward the body of a nerve cell. See also Protoplasm.

## DENDRITIC CELLS:

Patrolling immune system cells that may begin the HIV disease process by carrying the virus from the site of the infection to the lymph nodes, where other immune cells become infected. Dendritic cells travel through the body and bind to foreign invaders—such as HIV—especially in external tissues, such as the skin and the membranes of the gut, lungs and reproductive tract. They then ferry the foreign substance to the lymph nodes to stimulate T cells and initiate an immune response. In laboratory experiments, the dendritic cells that carry HIV also bind to CD4+ T cells, thereby allowing HIV to infect the CD4+ T cells. CD4+ T cells are the critical immune system cells targeted by HIV and depleted during HIV infection. See also CD4 (T4) or CD4+ Cells; Lymph Nodes; T Cells.

## D4T:

(Also known as Stavudine and Zerit). d4T is a dideoxynucleoside pyrimidine analog (2′3′-didehydro-3′-deoxythymidine). Like other nucleoside analogs, d4T inhibits HIV replication by inducing premature viral DNA chain termination. d4T has been approved for patients with advanced HIV infection intolerant to or failing other antiretroviral drugs. See also Nucleoside Analog.

## DIAGNOSIS:

The determination of the presence of a specific disease or infection, usually accomplished by evaluating clinical symptoms and laboratory tests.

**DIARRHEA:**
Uncontrolled, loose and frequent bowel movements. In the United States, almost all people with AIDS develop diarrhea at some time in the course of their disease. Severe or prolonged diarrhea can lead to weight loss and malnutrition. The excessive loss of fluid that may occur with AIDS-related diarrhea can be life-threatening. There are many possible causes of diarrhea in people who have AIDS. The most common infectious organism causing AIDS-related diarrhea include cytomegalovirus (CMV); the parasites *Cryptosporidium*, *Microsporidia* and *Giardia lamblia*; and the bacterium *Mycobacterium avium-inracellulare* (MAC). Other bacteria and parasites that cause diarrheal symptoms in otherwise healthy people may cause more severe, prolonged or recurrent diarrhea in people with HIV or AIDS. See also Cytomegalovirus; Giardiasis; Microsporidiosis; *Mycobacterium Avium* Complex.

**DIPLOPIA:**
Double vision.

**DISSEMINATED:**
Spread (of a disease) throughout the body.

**DIVISION OF AIDS TREATMENT RESEARCH INITIATIVE (DATRI):**
An organization established by the National Institute of Allergy and Infectious Diseases as a national network to test new therapies for HIV-infected persons. Its hallmark is the ability to rapidly conduct clinical trials and related research that evaluates new therapies and novel treatment approaches for those with HIV disease.

**DNA:**
(Deoxyribonucleic Acid). 1. The molecular chain found in genes within the nucleus of each cell, which carries the genetic information that enables cells to reproduce. 2. DNA is the principal constituent of chromosomes, the structures that transmit hereditary characteristics. The amount of DNA is constant for all typical cells of any given species

of plant or animal (including humans), regardless of the size or function of that cell. Each DNA molecule is a long, two-stranded chain made up of subunits, called nucleotides, containing a sugar (deoxyribose), a phosphate group and one of four nitrogenous bases: adenine (A), guanine (G), thymine (T) and cytosine (C). In 1953 J.D. Watson and F.H. Crick proposed that the strands, connected by hydrogen bonds between the bases, were coiled in a double helix. Adenine bonds only with thymine (A—T or T—A) and guanine only with cytosine (G—C or C—G). The complementarity of this bonding ensures that DNA can be replicated (i.e., that identical copies can be made in order to transmit genetic information to the next generation).

**DOMAIN:**
A region of a gene or gene product. See also Gene.

**DORMANCY:**
See Latency.

**DOSE-RANGING STUDY:**
A clinical trial in which two or more doses of an agent (such as a drug) are tested against each other to determine which dose works best and is least harmful. See also Clinical Trial.

**DOSE-RESPONSE RELATIONSHIP:**
The relationship between the dose of some agent (such as a drug), or the extent of exposure, and a physiological response. A dose-response effect means that as the dose increases so does the effect.

**DOUBLE-BLIND STUDY:**
A clinical trial design in which neither the participating individuals nor the study staff know which patients are receiving the experimental drug and which are receiving placebo or another therapy. Double-blind trials are thought to produce objective results, since the doctor's and patient's expectations about the experimental drug do not affect the outcome. See also Clinical Trial; Placebo.

## DRUG-DRUG INTERACTION:
A modification of the effect of a drug when administered with another drug. The effect may be an increase or a decrease in the action of either substance, or it may be an adverse effect that is not normally associated with either drug.

## DSMB:
See Data Safety and Monitoring Board.

## DYSPLASIA:
Any abnormal development of tissues or organs. In pathology, alteration in size, shape and organization of adult cells.

## DYSPNEA:
Difficult or labored breathing.

# E

**EFFICACY:**
(Of a drug or treatment). The maximum ability of a drug or treatment to produce a result regardless of dosage. A drug passes efficacy trials if it is effective at the dose tested and against the illness for which it is prescribed. In the procedure mandated by the Food and Drug Administration, phase II clinical trials gauge efficacy, phase III trials confirm it.

**ELISA:**
(Enzyme-Linked Immunosorbent Assay). A laboratory test to determine the presence of antibodies to HIV in the blood. A positive ELISA test generally is confirmed by the Western Blot test. See also Antibodies; Western Blot.

**EMPIRICAL:**
Based on experimental data, not on a theory.

**ENCEPHALITIS:**
A general term denoting inflammation of the brain.

**ENDEMIC:**
Pertaining to diseases associated with particular locales or population groups.

**ENDOGENOUS:**
Relating to or produced by the body.

**ENDOSCOPY:**
Viewing the inside of a body cavity (e.g., colon) with an endoscope, a device using flexible fiber optics.

**ENDOTOXIN:**
A toxin present inside a bacterial cell.

**END-STAGE DISEASE:**
Final period or phase in the course of a disease leading to a person's death.

**ENTERIC:**
Pertaining to the intestines.

**ENTERITIS:**
Inflammation of the intestine.

**ENV:**
A gene of HIV that codes for the protein gp160, the precursor of the envelope proteins gp120 and gp41. See also Gene.

**ENVELOPE:**
In virology, a protein covering that packages the virus's genetic information. The outer coat, or envelope, of HIV is composed of two layers of fat-like molecules called lipids taken from the membranes of human cells. Embedded in the envelope are numerous cellular protein, as well as mushroom-shaped HIV proteins that protrude from the surface. Each mushroom is thought to consist of a cap made of four glycoprotein molecules called gp120 and a stem consisting of four gp41 molecules embedded in the envelope. The virus uses these proteins to attach to and infect cells. See also Glycoprotein; gp41; gp120; Lipid.

**ENZYME:**
A protein that accelerates a specific chemical reaction without altering itself (i.e., a catalyst).

## EOSINOPHIL:

A type of white blood cell, called granulocyte, that can digest microorganisms. The granules can be stained by the acid dye, eosin, for microscopic examination.

## EPIDEMIC:

A disease that spreads rapidly through a demographic segment of the human population, such as everyone in a given geographic area, a military base, or similar population unit, or everyone of a certain age or sex, such as the children or women of a region. Epidemic diseases can be spread from person to person or from a contaminated source such as food or water.

## EPIDEMIOLOGIC SURVEILLANCE:

The ongoing and systematic collection, analysis and interpretation of data about a disease or health condition. As part of a surveillance system to monitor the HIV epidemic in the US, the CDC, in collaboration with state and local health departments, other federal agencies, blood collection agencies and medical research institutions, conducts standardized HIV seroprevalence surveys in designated subgroups in the US population. Collecting blood samples for the purpose of surveillance is called serosurveillance. See also Centers for Disease Control and Prevention; Seroprevalence;
Surveillance.

## EPIDEMIOLOGY:

The branch of medical science that deals with the incidence, distribution and control of a disease in a population.

## EPITHELIUM:

The covering of the internal and external organs of the body. Also the lining of vessels, body cavities, glands and organs. It consists of cells bound together by connective material and varies in the number of layers and the kinds of cells.

## EPITOPE:
A unique shape or marker carried on an antigen's surface that triggers a corresponding antibody response. See also Antibodies; Antigen.

## EPSTEIN-BARR VIRUS (EBV):
A herpes-like virus that causes one of the two kinds of mononucleosis (the other is caused by CMV). It infects the nose and throat and is contagious. EBV lies dormant in the lymph glands and has been associated with Burkitt's lymphoma and hairy leukoplakia. See also Burkitt's Lymphoma; Cytomegalovirus; Hairy Leukoplakia.

## ERYTHEMA:
Redness or inflammation of the skin or mucous membranes.

## ERYTHEMA MULTIFORME:
A skin disease characterized by papular (small, solid, usually conic elevation of the skin) or vesicular lesions (blisters), and reddening or discoloration of the skin often in concentric zones about the lesion. Erythema multiforme has been associated with many infections, collagen disease, drug sensitivities, allergies and pregnancy. A severe form of this condition is Stevens-Johnson Syndrome. See also Lesion; Stevens-Johnson Syndrome.

## ERYTHEMATOUS:
Red or reddened.

## ERYTHROCYTES:
Red blood cells whose major function is to carry oxygen to cells.

## ETIOLOGY:
The study or theory of the factors that cause disease.

## EXCLUSION/INCLUSION CRITERIA:
The medical or social standards determining whether a person may or may not be allowed to enter a clinical trial. For example, some trials

may not include people with chronic liver disease, or may exclude people with certain drug allergies; others may exclude men or women or only include people with a lowered T-cell count.

**EXOGENOUS:**
Developed or originating outside the body.

**EXOTOXIN:**
A toxic substance, made by bacteria, that is released outside the bacterial cell.

**EXPANDED ACCESS:**
A general term for methods of distributing experimental drugs to patients who are unable to participate in ongoing clinical trials and have no other treatment options. Specific types of expanded access mechanisms include parallel track, Treatment IND, and compassionate use. See also Investigational New Drug.

**EXPRESSION SYSTEM:**
In HIV vaccine production, cells into which an HIV gene has been inserted to produce desired HIV proteins.

# F

**FALLOPIAN TUBES:**

Part of the female reproductive system. A pair of ducts opening at one end into the uterus and at the other end into the peritoneal cavity, over the ovary. Each tube serves as a passage through which the ovum (egg) is carried to the uterus and through which spermatozoa (sperm) move toward the ovary. See also Ovary; Uterus.

**FDA:**

See Food and Drug Administration.

**FDCS:**

See Follicular Dendritic Cells.

**FOLIC ACID:**

A crystalline vitamin of the B complex that is used especially in the treatment of nutritional anemias. It occurs in green plants, fresh fruit, liver and yeast. Also called folacin, folate, vitamin $B_9$.

**FOLINIC ACID:**

Also called citrovorum factor. A metabolically active form of folic acid that has been used in cancer therapy to protect normal cells against methotrexate (a cancer chemotherapy agent). Also used to treat megaloblastic anemias. See also Folic Acid.

**FOLLICLE:**

A small anatomical cavity or deep narrow-mouthed depression; a small lymph node.

**FOLLICULAR DENDRITIC CELLS (FDCS):**

Cells found in the germinal centers of lymphoid organs. FDCs have thread-like tentacles that form a weblike network to trap invaders and present them to other cells of the immune system (for destruction). See also Lymphoid Organs.

## FOMITE:

An inanimate object that can harbor pathogenic microorganisms and thus serve as an agent of transmission of an infection.

## FOOD AND DRUG ADMINISTRATION (FDA):

The Public Health Service agency responsible for (among others) ensuring the safety and effectiveness of drugs, biologics, vaccines and medical devices used in the diagnosis, treatment and prevention of HIV infection, AIDS and AIDS-related opportunistic infections. The FDA also works with the blood banking industry to safeguard the nation's blood supply. See also Public Health Service.

## FUNCTIONAL ANTIBODY:

An antibody that binds to an antigen and has an effect. For example, neutralizing antibodies inactivate HIV or prevent it from infecting other cells. See also Antibodies; Antigen.

## FUNGUS:

1. A general term used to denote a class of microbes including mushrooms, yeasts and molds. 2. Fungi, which were once classified as plants, have since been reclassified as unmoving organisms that lack chlorophyll. Mycologists (scientists working with fungi) estimate that there are 100,000 species of fungi, ranging from baker's yeast to dermatophytes (fungi that cause ringworm and athlete's foot) to potentially invasive species such as *Candida albicans* and *Aspergillus*. As many as 150 of these organisms have now been linked to animal or human diseases.

# G

## GAMMA INTERFERON:

A T cell-derived stimulating substance that suppresses virus reproduction, stimulates other T cells and activates macrophage cells. See also Macrophage; T Cells.

## GANGLION:

A mass of nervous tissue, composed principally of nerve-cell bodies, usually lying outside the central nervous system.

## GASTROINTESTINAL:

Relating to the stomach and intestines.

## GENE:

1. A unit of DNA that carries information for the biosynthesis of a specific product (in the cell). 2. Ultimate unit by which inheritable characteristics are transmitted to succeeding generations in all living organisms. Genes are contained by, and arranged along the length of, the chromosome. The gene is composed of deoxyribonucleic acid (DNA). Each chromosome of each species has a definite number and arrangement of genes, which govern both the structure and metabolic functions of the cells and thus of the entire organism. They provide information for the synthesis of enzymes and other proteins and specify when these substances are to be made. Alteration of either gene number or arrangement can result in mutation (a change in the inheritable traits). See also DNA.

## GENETIC ENGINEERING:

Group of new research techniques that manipulate the DNA (genetic material) of cells. The gene-splicing technique, which produces recombinant DNA, is a method of transporting selected genes from one species to another. For example, in this technique, the genes, which are actually portions of molecules of DNA, are removed from the donor (insect, plant, mammal or other organism) and spliced into the genetic material of a virus; then the virus is allowed to infect recipient bacteria. In this way the bacteria become recipients of both viral and foreign genetic material. When the virus replicates within the bacteria, large quantities of the foreign as well as viral material are made.

### GENITOURINARY TRACT:

The system of organs comprising the organs concerned with the production and excretion of urine and those concerned with reproduction. Also called genitourinary system, urogenital system, urogenital tract.

### GENOME:

The complete set of genes in the chromosomes of each cell of a particular organism. See also Gene.

### GERMINAL CENTERS:

Structures within lymphoid tissues that contain FDCs in which immune responses are initiated. See also Follicular Dendritic Cells.

### GIARDIASIS:

A common protozoal infection of the small intestine spread via contaminated food and water and direct person-to-person contact.

### GLYCOPROTEIN:

A conjugated protein in which the nonprotein group is a carbohydrate (i.e., a sugar molecule); also called glucoprotein.

### GP41:

Glycoprotein 41, a protein embedded in the outer envelope of HIV. Plays a key role in HIV's infection of CD4+ T cells by facilitating the fusion of the viral and the cell membranes. See also CD4 (T4) or CD4+ Cells; Envelope.

## GP120:
Glycoprotein 120, a protein that protrudes from the surface of HIV and binds to CD4+ T cells. See also CD4 (T4) or CD4+ Cells.

## GP160:
Glycoprotein 160, a precursor of HIV envelope proteins gp41 and gp120.

## GRANULOCYTE:
A cell type of the immune system filled with granules of toxic chemicals that enable them to digest microorganisms. Basophils, neutrophils, and eosinophils are examples of granulocytes. See also Basophil; Eosinophil; Neutrophil.

## GUILLIAN-BARRÉ SYNDROME:
1. An acute febrile (i.e., with fever) polyneuritis. 2. An acute disease that produces bilateral (i.e., affecting the right and left sides of the body) weakness or paralysis, most commonly in the legs and feet. See also Polyneuritis.

# H

## HAIRY LEUKOPLAKIA:

A whitish, slightly raised lesion that appears on the side of the tongue. Thought to be related to Epstein-Barr virus infection, it was not observed before the HIV epidemic. See also Epstein-Barr Virus.

## HALF-LIFE:

The time required for half the amount of a drug to be eliminated from the body.

## HEALTH RESOURCES AND SERVICES ADMINISTRATION (HRSA):

A Public Health Service agency that administers (among others) education and training programs for health care providers and community service workers who care for AIDS patients. HRSA also administers programs to demonstrate how communities can organize their health care resources to develop an integrated, comprehensive system of care for those with AIDS and HIV infection. See also Public Health Service.

## HELPER/SUPPRESSOR RATIO:

(Of T cells). T cells are lymphocytes (white blood cells) that are formed in the thymus and are part of the immune system; they have been found to be abnormal in people with AIDS. The normal ratio of helper T cells (CD4+ cells) to suppressor T cells (CD8+ cells) is approximately 2:1. This becomes inverted in people with AIDS, but may be abnormal for a host of other temporary reasons. See also CD4 (T4) or CD4+ Cells; CD8 (T8) Cells; Lymphocyte; Thymus.

## HELPER T CELLS:

See CD4 (T4) or CD4+ Cells.

**HEMATOCRIT:**
A laboratory measurement that determines the percentage of packed red blood cells in a given volume of blood.

**HEMATOTOXIC:**
Poisonous to the blood or bone marrow.

**HEMOGLOBIN:**
The component of red blood cells that carries oxygen.

**HEMOLYSIS:**
The rupture of red blood cells.

**HEMOPHILIA:**
An inherited disease that prevents the normal clotting of blood.

**HEPATIC:**
Pertaining to the liver.

**HEPATITIS:**
An inflammation of the liver caused by certain viruses and other factors such as alcohol abuse, some medications and trauma. Although many cases of hepatitis are not a serious threat to health, the disease can become chronic and can sometimes lead to liver failure and death. There are four major types of viral hepatitis: (a) *hepatitis A,* caused by infection with the hepatitis A virus; (b) *hepatitis B*, caused by infection with the hepatitis B virus (HBV), which is most commonly passed on to a partner during intercourse, especially during anal sex, as well as through sharing drug needles; (c) *non-A, non-B hepatitis*, caused by the hepatitis C virus, which appears to be spread through sexual contact as well as through sharing drug needles (another type of non-A, non-B hepatitis is caused by the hepatitis E virus, principally spread through contaminated water) (d) *delta hepatitis* occurs only in people who are already infected with HBV and is caused by the HDV virus; most cases of delta hepatitis occur among people who are frequently exposed to

blood and blood products such as people with hemophilia. See also Hemophilia.

### HERPES SIMPLEX VIRUS I (HSV-I):

A virus that causes cold sores or fever blisters on the mouth or around the eyes, and can be transmitted to the genital region. The latent virus can be reactivated by stress, trauma, other infections or suppression of the immune system.

### HERPES SIMPLEX VIRUS II (HSV-II):

A virus causing painful sores of the anus or genitals that may lie dormant in nerve tissue. It can be reactivated to produce the symptoms. HSV-II may be transmitted to a neonate (newborn child) during birth from an infected mother, causing retardation and/or other serious complications. HSV-II is a precursor of cervical cancer. See also Cervical Cancer.

### HERPES VARICELLA ZOSTER VIRUS:

The varicella virus causes chicken pox in children and may reappear in adults as herpes zoster. Also called shingles, herpes zoster consists of very painful blisters on the skin that follow nerve pathways.

### HISTOCOMPATIBILITY TESTING:

A method of matching the self antigens on the tissues of a transplant donor with those of a recipient. The closer the match, the better the chance that the transplant will not be rejected. See also Human Leukocyte Antigens.

### HISTOPLASMOSIS:

A fungal infection, commonly of the lungs, caused by the fungus *Histoplasma capsulatum*. This fungus is commonly found in bird and/or bat droppings in the Ohio and Mississippi Valley region, the Caribbean Islands and in parts of the Northeast US. It is spread by breathing in the spores of the fungus. The most definitive test for the fungus has been from fungal stains and bone marrow cultures. Blood testing has proved to be less reliable. In areas where *H. capsulatum* is prevalent, 80 percent or more of the population has been exposed to infection through breathing in airborne spores produced by the fungus. People with severely damaged immune systems, such as those with AIDS, are vulnerable to a very serious disease known as progressive disseminated histoplasmosis. Nationwide, about 5 percent of people with AIDS have histoplasmosis, but in geographic areas where the fungus is common, people with AIDS are at high risk for disseminated histoplasmosis.

### HIV-1:
See Human Immunodeficiency Virus Type 1.

### HIV-2:
See Human Immunodeficiency Virus Type 2.

### HIV DISEASE:
Characterized by a gradual deterioration of immune function. During the course of infection, crucial immune cells called CD4+ T cells are disabled and killed, and their numbers progressively decline. CD4+ T cells play a crucial role in the immune response, signaling other cells in the immune system to perform their special functions. See also Acquired Immunodeficiency Syndrome; CD4 (T4) or CD4+ Cells; Human Immunodeficiency Virus Type 1.

### HIV-RELATED TUBERCULOSIS:
See Tuberculosis.

### HLA:
See Human Leukocyte Antigens.

### HODGKIN'S DISEASE:
See Lymphoma.

## HOMOLOGOUS:
Similar in appearance or structure, but not necessarily function.

## HOST:
A plant or animal harboring another organism.

## HOST FACTORS:
The body's potent mechanisms for containing HIV, including immune system cells called CD8+ T cells, which may prove more effective than any antiretro-viral drug in controlling HIV infection. See also Antiretroviral Agents; CD8 (T8) Cells.

## HRSA:
See Health Resources and Services Administration.

## HUMAN IMMUNODEFICIENCY VIRUS TYPE 1 (HIV-1):
1. The retrovirus isolated and recognized as the etiologic (i.e., causing or contributing to the cause of a disease) agent of AIDS. HIV-1 is classified as a lentivirus in a subgroup of retroviruses. See also Lentivirus; Retrovirus. 2. Most viruses and all bacteria, plants and animals have genetic codes made up of DNA, which uses RNA to build specific proteins. The genetic material of a retrovirus such as HIV is the RNA itself. HIV inserts its own RNA into the host cell's DNA, preventing the host cell from carrying out its natural functions and turning it into an HIV virus factory. See also DNA; Ribonucleic Acid.

## HUMAN IMMUNODEFICIENCY VIRUS TYPE 2 (HIV-2):
A virus closely related to HIV-1 that has been found to cause immune suppression. Most common in Africa.

## HUMAN LEUKOCYTE ANTIGENS (HLA):
Markers that identify cells as "self" and prevent the immune system from attacking them.

## HUMAN PAPILLOMA VIRUS (HPV):

A virus that is the cause of warts of the hands and feet, as well as lesions of the mucous membranes of the oral, anal and genital cavities. More than 50 types of HPV have been identified, some of which are associated with cancerous and precancerous conditions. The virus can be transmitted through sexual contact and is a precursor to cancer of the cervix. There is no specific cure for an HPV infection, but the virus often can be controlled by podophyllin (medicine derived from the roots of the plant *Podophyllum peltatum*) or interferon, and the warts can be removed by cryosurgery, laser treatment or conventional surgery. See also Cervical Cancer; Condyloma.

## HUMORAL IMMUNITY:

The branch of the immune system that relies primarily on antibodies. See also Antibodies; Cell-Mediated Immunity.

## HYBRID:

An offspring produced from mating plants or animals from different species, varieties or genotypes.

## HYBRIDOMA:

A hybrid cell produced by the fusion of an antibody-producing lymphocyte with a tumor cell. Hybridomas are used in the production of monoclonal antibodies. See also Hybrid; Lymphocyte; Monoclonal Antibodies.

## HYPERPLASIA:

Abnormal increase in the elements composing a part (as tissue cells).

## HYPOGAMMAGLOBULINEMIA:

Abnormally low levels of immunoglobulins. See also Antibodies.

## HYPOTHESIS:

A tentative statement or supposition that may then be tested through research.

**HYPOXIA:**

Reduction of oxygen supply to tissue.

# I

## IDIOPATHIC:
Without a known cause.

## IDIOTYPES:
The unique and characteristic parts of an antibody's variable region, which can themselves serve as antigens. See also Antibodies; Antigen.

## IHS:
See Indian Health Service.

## IMMUNE COMPLEX:
Clusters formed when antigens and antibodies bind together.

## IMMUNE DEFICIENCY:
A breakdown or inability of certain parts of the immune system to function, thus making a person susceptible to certain diseases that they would not ordinarily develop.

## IMMUNE RESPONSE:
The activity of the immune system against foreign substances.

## IMMUNE SYSTEM:
The complex functions of the body that recognize foreign agents or substances, neutralize them and recall the response later when confronted with the same challenge.

## IMMUNE THROMBOCYTOPENIC PURPURA (ITP):
Also Idiopathic Immune Thrombocytopenic Purpura. A condition in which the body produces antibodies against the platelets in the blood, which are cells responsible for blood clotting. ITP is very common in HIV-infected people. See also Antibodies; Platelets.

**IMMUNITY:**
A natural or acquired resistance to a specific disease. Im-munity may be partial or complete, long-lasting or temporary.

**IMMUNOCOMPETENT:**
1. Capable of developing an immune response. 2. Possessing a normal immune system.

**IMMUNODEFICIENCY:**
A deficiency of immune response or a disorder characterized by deficient immune response; classified as antibody (B cell), cellular (T cell), combined deficiency or phagocytic dysfunction disorders.

**IMMUNOGEN:**
A substance, also called an antigen, capable of provoking an immune response. See also Antigen.

**IMMUNOGENICITY:**
The ability of an antigen or vaccine to stimulate an immune response. See also Antigen.

**IMMUNOGLOBULIN:**
See Antibodies.

**IMMUNOLOGICAL SURVEILLANCE OR IMMUNOSURVEILLANCE:**
See Surveillance.

**IMMUNOMODULATOR:**
Any substance that influences the immune system.

**IMMUNOSTIMULANT:**
Any agent or substance that triggers or enhances the body's defense; also called immunopotentiators.

### IMMUNOSUPPRESSION:

A state of the body in which the immune system is damaged and does not perform its normal functions. Immunosuppression may be induced by drugs or result from certain disease processes, such as HIV infection. See also Immune System.

### IMMUNOTHERAPY:

Treatment aimed at reconstituting an impaired immune system. See also Immune System.

### IMMUNOTOXIN:

A plant or animal toxin (i.e., poison) that is attached to a monoclonal antibody and used to destroy a specific target cell. See also Antibiotic; Monoclonal Antibody.

### INCIDENCE:

The number of new cases occurring in a given population over a certain period of time.

### INCLUSION/EXCLUSION CRITERIA:

The medical or social standards determining whether a person may or may not be allowed to enter a clinical trial. For example, some trials may not allow people with chronic liver disease or with certain drug allergies; others may exclude men or women, or only include people with a lowered T-cell count.

### INCUBATION PERIOD:

The time interval between the initial exposure to infection and appearance of the first symptom or sign of disease.

### IND:

See Investigational New Drug.

## INDIAN HEALTH SERVICE (IHS):

A Public Health Service agency providing a comprehensive health service delivery system for American Indians and Alaska Natives. See also Public Health Service.

## INFECTION:

The state or condition in which the body (or part of the body) is invaded by an infectious agent (e.g., a bacterium, fungus or virus), which multiplies and produces an injurious effect (active infection). As related to HIV: Infection typically begins when HIV encounters a CD4+ cell. The HIV surface protein gp120 binds tightly to the CD4 molecule on the cell's surface. The membranes of the virus and the cell fuse, a process governed by gp41, another surface protein. The viral core, containing HIV's RNA, proteins and enzymes, is released into the cell. See CD4 (T4) or CD4+ Cells; gp41; gp120.

## INFECTIOUS:

Capable of being transmitted by infection, with or without actual contact. See also Infection.

## INFORMED CONSENT:

Type of protection available to people considering entering a drug trial. Before entering the trial, participants must sign a consent form that contains an explanation of: (a) why the research is being done, (b) what researchers want to accomplish, (c) what will be done during the trial and for how long, (d) what risks are in the trial, (e) what benefits can be expected from the trial, (f) what other treatments are available, and (g) the participant's right to leave the trial at any time. See also Clinical Trial.

## INOCULATION:

The introduction of a substance (inoculum; e.g., a vaccine, serum or virus) into the body to produce or to increase immunity to the disease or condition associated with the substance. See also Vaccine.

## INSTITUTIONAL REVIEW BOARD (IRB):

1. A committee of physicians, statisticians, community advocates and others that ensures that a clinical trial is ethical and that the rights of study participants are protected. All clinical trials in the United States must be approved by an IRB before they begin. See also Clinical Trial. 2. Every institution that conducts or supports biomedical or behavioral research involving human subjects must, by federal regulation, have an IRB that initially approves and periodically reviews the research so as to protect the rights of human subjects.

## INTEGRASE:

An HIV enzyme used by the virus to integrate its genetic material into the host cell's DNA. See also DNA; Enzyme.

## INTEGRATION:

The process by which the different parts of an organism are made a functional and structural whole, especially through the activity of the nervous system and of hormones. As related to HIV: The process by which the viral DNA migrates to the cell's nucleus, where it is spliced into the host's DNA with the help of viral integrase. Once incorporated, HIV DNA is called the provirus and is duplicated together with the cell's genes every time the cell divides. Recent reports suggest that HIV's DNA also can integrate into the DNA of nondividing cells such as macro-phages and brain and nerve cells. See also Integrase; Macrophage.

## INTENT TO TREAT:

Analysis of clinical trial results that includes all data from patients in the groups to which they were randomized (i.e., assigned through random distribution) even if they never received the treatment. See also Clinical Trial.

## INTERFERON:

A general term used to describe a family of 20–25 proteins that cause a cell to become resistant to a wide variety of viruses. They are produced by cells infected by almost any virus.

## INTERLEUKIN-2 (IL-2):

One of a family of molecules that control the growth and function of many types of lymphocytes. Interleukin-2 is an immune system protein produced in the body by T cells. It has potent effects on the proliferation, differentiation and activity of a number of immune system cells, including T cells, B cells and natural killer cells. Commercially, IL-2 is produced by recombinant DNA technology and is approved by the Food and Drug Administration for the treatment of metastatic renal (i.e., kidney) cell cancer. Studies have shown that in the test tube, addition of IL-2 can improve some of the immunologic functions that are abnormal in HIV-infected patients. In addition, IL-2 is a growth factor for T cells, causing them to increase in number. In a clinical study with IL-2, it was found that in a small number of HIV-infected patients, IL-2 boosted levels of CD4+ T cells (i.e., the infection-fighting white blood cells normally destroyed during HIV infection) for more than two years, a far longer time than typically seen with currently available anti-HIV drugs. See also Biotechnology; B Lymphocytes; Genetic Engineering; Killer T Cells; Lymphocyte; T Cells.

## INTERSTITIAL:

Relating to or situated in the small, narrow spaces between tissues or parts of an organ.

## INTRAMUSCULAR:

Injected directly into a muscle.

## INTRATHECAL:

Injected into the fluid surrounding the spinal cord.

**INTRAVENOUS (IV):**
Of or pertaining to the inside of a vein, as of a thrombus, or an injection, infusion or catheter.

**INTRAVITREAL:**
Within the eye.

**INVESTIGATIONAL NEW DRUG (IND):**
The status of an experimental drug after the Food and Drug Administration agrees that it can be tested in people.

**IN VITRO:**
("In glass"). An artificial environment created outside a living organism (e.g., a test tube or culture plate) used in experimental research to study a disease or process.

**IN VIVO:**
("In life"). Studies conducted within a living organism (e.g., animal or human studies).

**IRB:**
See Institutional Review Board.

**ISOLATE:**
An individual (as a spore or a single organism), viable part of an organism (as a cell) or a strain that has been isolated (as from diseased tissue, contaminated water or the air). Also, a pure culture produced from such an isolate. A particular strain of HIV taken from a patient.

**ITP:**
See Immune Thrombocytopenic Purpura.

# K

## KAPOSI'S SARCOMA:

1. A previously uncommon form of cancer that attacks the connective tissue, bones, cartilage and muscles of the body. The cancer may spread and also attack the eyes. If the cancerous area is near the surface of the skin, lesions inches in length may develop. This disease was initially seen only in elderly men and natives of Central Africa. Experimental work has shown that the AIDS-related Kaposi's sarcoma and the Central African variety respond differently to some types of medications. Radiotherapy and chemotherapy are usually recommended. 2. A type of cancer characterized by abnormal growths of blood vessels that develop into purplish or brown lesions. It is suspected that the cause of Kaposi's sarcoma is a newly found herpes virus.

## KARNOFSKY SCORE:

A subjective score between 0–100, assigned by a physician to describe a patient's ability to perform common tasks.

## KILLER T CELLS:

Killer cells infected with HIV or other viruses or transformed by cancer. Also known as cytotoxic T cells (or cytotoxic T lymphocytes). See also Null Cell; T Cells.

## KUPFFER CELLS:

Specialized macrophages in the liver. See also Macrophage.

# L

## LAI:
A group of closely related HIV isolates that includes the LAV, IIIB and BRU strains of HIV. Used in HIV vaccine development. See also Isolate.

## LAK CELLS:
Lymphocytes transformed in the laboratory into lymphokine activated killer cells, which attack tumor cells. See also Lymphocyte; Lymphokines.

## LANGERHANS CELLS:
Dendritic cells in the skin that pick up an antigen and transport it to the lymph nodes. See also Antigen; Dendritic Cells; Lymph Nodes.

## LAS:
See Lymphadenopathy Syndrome.

## LATENCY:
The period when an organism (i.e., a virus or a bacterium) is in the body and not producing any ill effects. See also Clinical Latency.

## LAV:
Lymphadenopathy Associated Virus (see Human Immunodeficiency Virus Type I).

## LENTIVIRUS:
"Slow" virus characterized by a long interval between infection and the onset of symptoms. HIV is a lentivirus as is the simian immunodeficiency virus (SIV), which infects nonhuman primates. See also Simian Immunodeficiency Virus.

## LESION:
A general term to describe an area of altered tissue (e.g., the infected patch or sore in a skin disease).

## LEUKOCYTES:
All white blood cells.

## LEUKOPENIA:
A decrease in the number of white blood cells. The threshold value for leukopenia is usually taken as less than 5000 white blood cells per cubic millimeter of blood.

## LIP:
See Lymphoid Interstitial Pneumonitis.

## LIPID:
Any of a group of fats and fat-like compounds, including sterols, fatty acids and many other substances.

## LIPOSOMES:
A spherical particle in an aqueous (watery) medium (e.g., inside a cell) formed by a lipid bilayer enclosing an aqueous compartment. See also Lipid.

## LONG TERMINAL REPEAT SEQUENCE (LTR):
A component of the AIDS genome. See also Genome.

## LONG-TERM NON-PROGRESSORS:
Individuals who are HIV-infected for seven or more years, have stable CD4+ T cell counts of 600 or more cells per cubic millimeter of blood, no HIV-related diseases and no previous antiretroviral therapy. Data suggest that this phenomenon is associated with the maintenance of the integrity of the lymphoid tissues and with less virus-trapping in the lymph nodes than seen in other HIV-infected individuals.

## LTR:

See Long Terminal Repeat Sequence.

## LUMBAR:

Of, relating to or constituting the loins or the vertebrae between the thoracic vertebrae and the sacrum region. The sacrum is the triangular bone made up of five fused vertebrae and forming the posterior section of the pelvis. The thorax is the part of the human body between the neck and the diaphragm, partially encased by the ribs and containing the heart and lungs; the chest.

## LUMBAR PUNCTURE:

A procedure in which fluid from the subarachnoid space in the lumbar region is tapped for examination. Also known as spinal tap. See also Lumbar; Subarachnoid Space.

## LYMPH:

A transparent, slightly yellow fluid that carries lymphocytes. Lymph is derived from tissue fluids collected from all parts of the body and is returned to the blood via lymphatic vessels. See also Lymphatic Vessels; Lymphocyte.

## LYMPHADENOPATHY SYNDROME (LAS):

Swollen, firm and possibly tender lymph nodes. The cause may range from an infection such as HIV, the flu, mononucleosis or lymphoma (cancer of the lymph nodes). See also Lymph Nodes.

## LYMPHATIC VESSELS:

A bodywide network of channels, similar to the blood vessels, that transport lymph to the immune organs and into the bloodstream. See also Lymph.

## LYMPH NODES:

Small, bean-sized organs of the immune system, distributed widely throughout the body. Lymph fluid is filtered through the lymph nodes in which all types of lymphocytes take up temporary residence. Antigens that enter the body find their way into lymph or blood and are filtered out by the lymph nodes or spleen respectively, for attack by the immune system. See also Antigen; Lymphocyte.

**LYMPHOCYTE:**
A white blood cell. Present in the blood, lymph and lymphoid tissue. See also B Lymphocytes; Lymph; T Cells.

**LYMPHOID INTERSTITIAL PNEUMONITIS (LIP):**
A form of pneumonia that involves the lower lobes (of the lungs) with extensive alveolar infiltration by mature lymphocytes, plasma cells and histiocytes. LIP is associated with AIDS, dysproteinemia and other conditions. See also Alveolar; Lymphocyte; Macrophage.

**LYMPHOID ORGANS:**
Include tonsils, adenoids, lymph nodes, spleen and other tissues. Act as the body's filtering system, trapping invaders (i.e., foreign particles from bacteria, viruses, etc.) and presenting them to squadrons of immune cells that congregate there. Within these lymphoid tissues, immune activity is concentrated in regions called germinal centers, where the thread-like tentacles of follicular dendritic cells (FDCs) form networks that trap invaders. See also Follicular Dendritic Cells; Lymph Nodes.

**LYMPHOKINES:**
1. Products of the lymphatic cells that stimulate the production of disease-fighting agents and the activities of other lymphatic cells. Among the lymphokines are gamma interferon and interleukin-2. See also Gamma Interferon; Interleukin-2. 2. Nonanti-body mediators of immune responses, released by activated lymphocytes. See also Immune Response; Lymphocyte.

## LYMPHOMA:

Cancer of the lymphoid tissues. Lymphomas are often described as being large or small cell types, cleaved or noncleaved, diffuse or nodular. The different types often have different prognoses (i.e., prospect of survival or recovery). Some of these lymphomas are named after the physicians who first described them (e.g., Burkitt's lymphoma, Hodgkin's disease). Lymphomas can also be referred to by the organ where they are active such as CNS lymphomas, which are in the central nervous system, and GI lymphomas, which are in the gastrointestinal tract. The types of lymphomas most commonly associated with HIV infection are called non-Hodgkin's lymphomas or B cell lymphomas. In these types of cancers, certain cells of the lymphatic system grow abnormally. They divide rapidly, growing into tumors.

## LYSIS:

Rupture and destruction of a cell.

## MACROPHAGE:

A large immune cell that devours invading pathogens and other intruders. Stimulates other immune cells by presenting them with small pieces of the invader. Macrophages can harbor large quantities of HIV without being killed, acting as reservoirs of the virus.

## MAGNETIC RESONANCE IMAGING (MRI):

Medical imaging that uses radiofrequency radiation as its source. MRI is a noninvasive diagnostic technique that can provide information on the form and function of internal tissues and organs of the body.

## MAJOR HISTOCOMPATIBILITY COMPLEX (MHC):

A group of genes that control aspects of the immune response. The products of these genes, the histocompatibility antigens, are present on every cell of the body and serve as markers to distinguish self from nonself cells. See also Antigen; Histocompatibility Testing.

## MALABSORPTION SYNDROME:

Decreased intestinal absorption resulting in loss of appetite, muscle pain and weight loss.

## MALAISE:

A generalized, nonspecific feeling of discomfort.

## MAST CELL:

A granulocyte found in tissue. The contents of the mast cells, along with those of basophils, are responsible for the symptoms of allergy. See also Basophil; Granulocyte.

## MEAN:
The arithmetic average, or the sum of all the values divided by the number of values.

## MEDIAN:
The middle number in a sequence of numbers, taken as the average of the two middle numbers when the sequence has an even number of numbers (e.g., 4 is the median of 1, 3, 4, 8, 9).

## MEMORY CELLS:
A subset of T lymphocytes that have been exposed to specific antigens and can then proliferate (i.e., reproduce) on subsequent immune system encounters with the same antigen. See also Antigen; T Cells.

## MESSENGER RNA:
Also referred to as mRNA. An RNA (ribonucleic acid) that carries the genetic code for a particular protein from the nuclear DNA (i.e., the DNA in the cell's nucleus) to a ribosome in the cytoplasm and acts as a template, or pattern, for the formation of that protein. See also Cytoplasm; Ribosome.

## METABOLISM:
The sum of the processes by which a particular substance is handled (as by assimilation and incorporation, or by detoxification and excretion) in the living body.

## METABOLITE:
Any substance produced by metabolism or by a metabolic process. See also Metabolism.

## METASTASIS:
Transfer of a disease-producing agent (e.g., cancer cells or bacteria) from an original site of disease to another part of the body with development of a similar lesion in the new location (e.g., spread of cancer from an original site to other sites in the body).

## MHC:
See Major Histocompatibility Complex.

## MICROBES:
Microscopic living organisms, including bacteria, protozoa and fungi.

## MICROBICIDE:
An agent (e.g., a chemical or antibiotic) that destroys microbes. See also Microbes.

## MICROENCAPSULATED:
Surrounded by a thin layer of protection. A means of protecting a drug or vaccine from rapid breakdown.

## MICROSPORIDIOSIS:
Disease resulting from infection with a protozoal pathogen from the *Microsporida* order. See also Pathogen; Protozoa.

## MN:
A strain of HIV used in vaccine development.

## MOLECULE:
The smallest particle of a compound that has all the chemical properties of that compound. Molecules are made up of two or more atoms, either of the same element or of two or more different elements. Ionic compounds, such as common salt, are made up not of molecules, but of ions arranged in a crystalline structure. Unlike ions, molecules carry no electrical charge. Molecules differ in size and molecular weight as well as in structure.

## MOLLUSCUM CONTAGIOSUM:
A disease of the skin and mucous membranes caused by a poxvirus. It is characterized by scattered flesh-toned white papules. The disease most frequently occurs in children and adults with impaired immune

response. It is transmitted from person to person by direct or indirect contact and lasts up to three years.

**MONOCLONAL ANTIBODIES:**
Antibodies produced by a hybridoma or antibody-producing cell source for a specific antigen. Monoclonal antibodies are useful as a tool for identifying specific protein molecules. See also Antibodies; Antigen; Hybridoma.

**MONOCYTE:**
A large white blood cell that ingests microbes or other cells and foreign particles. When a monocyte enters tissues, it develops into a macrophage. See also Macrophage.

**MONOVALENT VACCINE:**
A vaccine that is specific for only one antigen. See also Antigen.

**MRI:**
See Magnetic Resonance Imaging.

**MUCOCUTANEOUS:**
Anything that concerns or pertains to mucous membranes and the skin (e.g., mouth, vagina, lips, anal area). See also Mucous Membrane.

**MUCOSA:**
See Mucous Membrane.

**MUCOSAL IMMUNITY:**
Resistance to infection across the mucous membranes. Dependent on immune cells and antibodies present in the lining of the urogenital tract, gastrointestinal tract and other parts of the body exposed to the outside world. See also Antibodies; Genitourinary Tract; Mucous Membrane.

## MUCOUS MEMBRANE:

A moist layer of tissue that lines body cavities or passages that have an opening to the external world (e.g., the lining of the mouth, nostrils or vagina).

## MUTATION:

In biology, a sudden change in a gene or unit of hereditary material that results in a new inheritable characteristic. In higher animals and many higher plants, a mutation may be transmitted to future generations only if it occurs in germ—or sex cell—tissue; body cell mutations cannot be inherited. Changes within the chemical structure of single genes may be induced by exposure to radiation, temperature extremes and certain chemicals. The term mutation may also be used to include losses or rearrangements of segments of chromosomes, the long strands of genes. Drugs such as colchicine double the normal number of chromosomes in a cell by interfering with cell division. Mutation, which can establish new traits in a population, is important in evolution. As related to HIV: HIV mutates rapidly. During the course of HIV disease, viral strains may emerge in an infected individual that differ widely in their ability to infect and kill different cell types, as well as in their rate of replication. Strains of HIV from patients with advanced disease appear to be more virulent and infect more cell types than strains obtained earlier from the same individual. See also Gene.

## MYCOBACTERIUM:

Any bacterium of the genus *Mycobacterium* or a closely related genus.

## MYCOBACTERIUM AVIUM COMPLEX (MAC):

1. A common opportunistic infection caused by two very similar mycobacterial organisms, *Mycobacterium avium* and *Mycobacterium intracellulare*. 2. A bacterial infection that can be localized (limited to a specific organ or area of the body) or disseminated throughout the body. It is a life-threatening disease, although new therapies offer promise for both prevention and treatment. MAC disease is extremely

rare in people who are not infected with HIV. See also Opportunistic Infection.

**MYCOPLASMA:**
1. Smallest free-living organisms known to infect humans. Mycoplasma cause a variety of illnesses, especially of the lungs and sexual organs. 2. Any microorganism of the genus *Mycoplasma,* also called *pleuropneumonia-like* organism.

**MYCOSIS:**
Any disease caused by a fungus. See also Fungus.

**MYELIN:**
A substance that sheathes nerve cells, acting as an electric insulator that facilitates the conduction of nerve impulses.

**MYELOSUPPRESSION:**
Impairment of the blood cell–producing function of the bone marrow.

**MYELOTOXIC:**
Destructive to bone marrow.

# N

## NATIONAL AIDS CLEARINGHOUSE:

See CDC National AIDS Clearinghouse.

## NATIONAL CANCER INSTITUTE (NCI):

An NIH institute with the overall mission of conducting and supporting research, training and disseminating health information with respect to the causes, diagnosis and treatment of cancer. NCI also performs these functions for HIV infections and associated diseases. See also National Institutes of Health.

## NATIONAL INSTITUTE OF ALLERGY AND INFECTIOUS DISEASES (NIAID):

An NIH institute that conducts and supports research to study the causes of allergic, immunologic and infectious diseases, and to develop better means of preventing, diagnosing and treating illnesses. NIAID is responsible for the federally funded, national basic research program in AIDS. See also National Institutes of Health.

## NATIONAL INSTITUTE OF CHILD HEALTH AND HUMAN DEVELOPMENT (NICHD):

An NIH institute that conducts and supports research on the reproductive, developmental and behavioral processes that determine the health of children, adults, families and populations. Thus, NICHD supports clinical research related to the transmission of HIV from infected mothers to their offspring, the progression of disease in HIV-infected infants and children, and the testing of potential therapies and preventatives for this population. See also National Institutes of Health.

## NATIONAL INSTITUTES OF HEALTH (NIH):

A multi-institute agency of the Public Health Service, NIH is the federal focal point for health research. It conducts research in its own laboratories and supports research in universities, medical schools, hospitals and research institutions throughout this country and abroad. See also Public Health Service.

### NATIONAL LIBRARY OF MEDICINE (NLM):

An NIH institute, NLM is one of three US national libraries. It is the world's largest research library in a single scientific and professional field (i.e., medicine). NLM provides (among others) electronic and print information services relating to HIV/AIDS, including AIDSLINE, AIDSTRIALS, AIDSDRUGS and the AIDS Bibliography. See also AIDS Bibliography; AIDSDRUGS; AIDSLINE; AIDSTRIALS; National Institutes of Health.

### NATURAL HISTORY STUDY:

Study of the natural development of something (such as an organism or a disease) over a period of time.

### NATURAL KILLER CELLS:

(NK cells). A type of lymphocyte that does not carry the markers to be B cells or T cells. Like cytotoxic T cells, they attack and kill tumor cells and protect against a wide variety of infectious microbes. They are "natural" killers because they do not need additional stimulation or need to recognize a specific antigen in order to attack and kill. Persons with immunodeficiences such as those caused by HIV infection have a decrease in "natural" killer cell activity. See also Antigen; B Lymphocytes; Cytotoxic; Lymphocyte; Null Cell; T Cells.

### NCI:

See National Cancer Institute.

### NEBULIZED:

See Aerosolized.

## NECROLYSIS:
Shedding of surface components of tissue, such as cells from internal body surfaces, due to death of a portion of tissue.

## NEF:
One of the regulatory genes of the HIV virus. Three HIV regulatory genes—tat, rev and nef—and three so-called auxiliary genes—vif, vpr and vpu—contain information necessary for the production of proteins that control the virus's ability to infect a cell, produce new copies of the virus or cause disease. See also rev; tat.

## NEONATAL:
Concerning the first four weeks of life after birth.

## NEOPLASM:
An abnormal and uncontrolled growth of tissue; a tumor.

## NEPHROTOXIC:
Poisonous to the kidneys.

## NEURALGIA:
A sharp, shooting pain along a nerve pathway.

## NEUROLOGICAL COMPLICATIONS OF AIDS:
See Central Nervous System (CNS) Damage.

## NEUROPATHY:
The name given to a group of disorders involving nerves. Symptoms range from a tingling sensation or numbness in the toes and fingers to paralysis. It is estimated that 35 percent of people with HIV disease have some form of neuropathy. A "peripheral neuropathy" refers to the peripheral nerves outside the spinal cord.

**NEUTRALIZATION:**
The process by which an antibody binds to specific antigens, thereby "neutralizing" the microorganism. See also Antibodies; Antigen.

**NEUTRALIZING ANTIBODY:**
An antibody that keeps a virus from infecting a cell, usually by blocking receptors on the cell or the virus. See also Antibodies; Receptor.

**NEUTRALIZING DOMAIN:**
The section of the HIV envelope protein gp120 that elicits antibodies with neutralizing activities. See also Antibodies; gp120.

**NEUTROPENIA:**
An abnormal decrease in the number of neutrophils (the most common type of white blood cells) in the blood. The decrease may be relative or absolute. Neutropenia is associated with acute leukemia, infection, rheumatoid arthritis and other conditions.

**NEUTROPHIL:**
Also called polymorphonuclear neutrophil (PMN). A white blood cell that plays a central role in defense of a host against infection. Neutrophils engulf and kill foreign microorganisms.

**NIAID:**
See National Institute of Allergy and Infectious Diseases.

**NICHD:**
See National Institute of Child Health and Human Development.

**NIH:**
See National Institutes of Health.

**NLM:**
See National Library of Medicine.

## NON-HODGKIN'S LYMPHOMA:

See Lymphoma.

## NSAID:

Nonsteroidal anti-inflammatory (i.e., counteracting inflammation) drug.

## NUCLEIC ACID:

Organic substance, found in all living cells, in which the hereditary information is stored and from which it can be transferred. Nucleic acid molecules are long chains that generally occur in combination with proteins. The two chief types are DNA (deoxyribonucleic acid), found mainly in cell nuclei, and RNA (ribonucleic acid), found mostly in cytoplasm. Each nucleic acid chain is composed of subunits called nucleotides, each containing a sugar, a phosphate group, and one of four bases: adenine (symbolized A), guanine (G), cytosine (C) and thymine (T). RNA contains the sugar ribose instead of deoxyribose and the base uracil (U) instead of thymine. The specific sequences of nucleotides constitute the cell's genetic information: Each three-nucleotide DNA sequence specifies one particular amino acid. The long sequences of DNA nucleotides thus correspond to the sequences of amino acids in the cell's proteins. In order to be expressed as protein, the genetic information is carried to the protein-synthesizing machinery of the cell, usually in the cell cytoplasm. Forms of RNA mediate this process. DNA not only provides information, but also specifies its own exact replication. The cell replicates its DNA by making a complementary copy of its exact nucleotide sequence: T for every A, C for every G, G for every C, A for every T. Although the triplet nucleotide code seems to be universal, the actual sequences of the nucleotides vary according to the species and individual. See also Gene; Genetic Engineering; Mutation.

## NUCLEOLI:

Bodies in the nucleus that become enlarged during protein synthesis and contain the DNA template for ribosomal RNA. See also Ribonucleic Acid; Ribosome.

## NUCLEOSIDE ANALOG:

Nucleosides are related to nucleotides, the subunits of nucleic acids; however, they do not carry the phosphate groups of the nucleotides. Nucleoside analogs generally are synthetic compounds similar to one of the components of DNA or RNA; a general type of antiviral drug (e.g., acyclovir and AZT). See also Acyclovir; AZT; Nucleic Acid.

## NUCLEUS:

1. The central controlling body within a living cell, usually a spherical unit enclosed in a membrane and containing genetic codes for maintaining the life systems of the organism and for issuing commands for growth and reproduction. 2. The nucleus of a cell is an organelle (i.e., a cellular organ) that is essential to such cell functions as reproduction and protein synthesis. It is composed of nuclear sap and a nucleoprotein-rich network from which chromosomes and nucleoli arise and is enclosed in a definite membrane. See also Nucleoli.

## NULL CELL:

A lymphocyte that develops in the bone marrow and lacks the characteristic surface markers of the B and T lymphocytes. Null cells represent a small proportion of the lymphocyte population. Stimulated by the presence of antibody, null cells can attack certain cellular targets directly and are known as "natural killer" or NK cells. See also Lymphocyte.

# O

## OCULAR:
Pertaining to the eye.

## OPEN-LABEL TRIAL:
A clinical trial in which doctors and participants know which drug or vaccine is being administered. See also Clinical Trial.

## OPPORTUNISTIC INFECTION:
1. An illness caused by an organism that usually does not cause disease in a person with a normal immune system. People with advanced HIV infection suffer opportunistic infections of the lungs, brain, eyes and other organs. 2. Opportunistic infections common in AIDS patients include *Pneumocystis carinii* pneumonia, Kaposi's sarcoma, shigellosis, histoplasmosis and other parasitic, viral, and fungal infections, and some types of cancers. See also Histoplasmosis; Kaposi's Sarcoma; *Pneumocystis carinii* Pneumonia.

## OROPHARYNGEAL:
Relating to that division of the pharynx between the soft palate and the epiglottis. Pharynx is a tube that connects the mouth and nasal passages with the esophagus, the connection to the stomach. Epiglottis is a thin, valvelike structure that covers the glottis, the opening of the upper part of the larynx (the part of the throat containing the vocal cords), during swallowing.

## OVARY:
Part of the female reproductive system. One of a pair of female gonads (a gamete-producing gland) found on each side of the lower abdomen, beside the uterus, in a fold of the broad ligament. At ovulation, an egg is extruded from a follicle on the surface of the ovary under the stimulation of certain hormones.

# P

## P24:

1. Within the envelope of the HIV virus is a bullet-shaped core made of another protein, p24, that surrounds the viral RNA. 2. The p24 antigen test looks for the presence of this protein in a patient's blood. 3. A positive result for the p24 antigen suggests active HIV replication. p24 found in the peripheral blood is thought to also correlate with the amount of virus in the peripheral blood. It is believed that there are measurable levels of p24 when first infected with the virus after which there is a strong antibody response to p24 in early disease. Low or unmeasurable levels of p24 may indicate that the virus is in a dormant stage. Spikes in p24 levels may indicate that HIV has begun active replication.

## PALLIATIVE:

A treatment that provides symptomatic relief, but not a cure.

## PANCREAS:

A gland situated near the stomach that secretes a digestive fluid into the intestine through one or more ducts and also secretes the hormone insulin.

## PANCREATITIS:

Inflammation of the pancreas that can produce severe pain and debilitating illness. See also Pancreas.

## PANCYTOPENIA:

Deficiency of all cell elements of the blood.

## PANDEMIC:

A disease prevalent throughout an entire country, continent or the whole world. See also Epidemic.

## PAP SMEAR:
A method for the early detection of cancer and other abnormalities of the female genital tract, especially of the cervix and uterus, employing exfoliated cells (cells that have been shed into vaginal fluid) and a special staining technique for microscopic examination that differentiates diseased tissue. Also known as Papanicolaou Smear after George Papanicolaou, the American cytologist who developed this method and published it in 1943. See also Cervix; Uterus.

## PAPILLOMA:
1. A benign tumor (as a wart or condyloma) resulting from an overgrowth of epithelial tissue on papillae of vascularized connective tissue (as of the skin). 2. An epithelial tumor caused by a virus. See also Condyloma; Epithelium.

## PARALLEL TRACK:
A system of distributing experimental drugs to patients who are unable to participate in ongoing clinical efficacy trials and have no other treatment options. See also Clinical Trial.

## PARASITE:
A plant or animal that lives and feeds on or within another living organism; does not necessarily cause disease.

## PARENCHYMA:
The tissue of an organ (as distinguished from supporting or connective tissue).

## PARENTERAL:
Not in or through the digestive system. For example, parenteral can pertain to blood being drawn from a vein in the arm or introduced into that vein via a transfusion (intravenous), or to injection of medications or vaccines through the skin (subcutaneous) or into the muscle (intramuscular).

**PARESTHESIA:**
Any subjective sensation, experienced as numbness, tingling or a "pins-and-needles" feeling.

**PATHOGEN:**
Any disease-producing microorganism or material.

**PATHOGENESIS:**
The origin and development of a disease.

**PBMC:**
See Peripheral Blood Mononuclear Cell.

**PCP:**
See *Pneumocystis carinii* Pneumonia.

**PCR:**
See Polymerase Chain Reaction.

**PEER REVIEW:**
The process by which new scientific or medical findings, announced by one researcher, are reviewed by other scientists or physicians before these findings are published.

**PELVIC INFLAMMATORY DISEASE (PID):**
A term used to describe infections of the uterus, the fallopian tubes and the ovaries. PID is usually the result of untreated sexually transmitted disease, primarily chlamydia or gonorrhea. See also Fallopian Tubes; Ovary; Uterus.

**PENTAMIDINE:**
An approved antiprotozoal drug used for the treatment and prevention of *Pneumocystis carinii* pneumonia (PCP) infection. It can be delivered intravenously or intramuscularly or inhaled as an aerosol. Aerosolized pentamidine is approved for the prophylaxis of PCP in HIV-positive

individuals with CD4+ counts below 200 per cubic millimeter or for those with prior episodes of PCP. The drug is also known under the names Pentam and NebuPent. See also *Pneumocystis carinii* Pneumonia.

**PEPTIDE:**
(Also polypeptide). Biochemical formed by the linkage of up to about 50 amino acids to form a chain. Longer chains are called proteins. The amino acids are coupled by a peptide bond, a special linkage in which the nitrogen atom of one amino acid binds to the carboxyl carbon atom of another. Many peptides, such as the hormones vasopressin and ACTH, have physiological or antibacterial activity. See also Amino Acids.

**PERIANAL:**
Around the anus.

**PERINATAL:**
Events that occur at or around the time of birth.

**PERIPHERAL BLOOD MONONUCLEAR CELL (PBMC):**
Cells in the bloodstream with one nucleus. See also Nucleus.

**PERSISTENT GENERALIZED LYMPHADENOPATHY (PGL):**
Chronic, diffuse, noncancerous lymph node enlargement. Typically it has been found in those with immune system disturbances who develop frequent and persistent bacterial, viral and fungal infections.

**PGL:**
See Persistent Generalized Lymphadenopathy.

**PHA:**
See Phytohemagglutinin.

## PHAGOCYTE:

A cell that is able to ingest and destroy foreign matter, including bacteria.

## PHAGOCYTOSIS:

The process of ingesting and destroying a virus or other foreign matter by phagocyte. See also Macrophage; Monocyte.

## PHARMACOKINETICS:

The processes (in a living organism) of absorption, distribution, metabolism and excretion of a drug or vaccine.

## PHS:

See Public Health Service.

## PHYTOHEMAGGLUTININ (PHA):

A plant chemical used to stimulate the multiplication of white blood cells.

## PITUITARY GLAND:

Small, oval endocrine gland that lies at the base of the brain. It is called the master gland because the other endocrine glands depend on its secretions for stimulation. The pituitary has two distinct lobes, anterior and posterior. The anterior lobe secretes at least six hormones: human growth hormone, which stimulates overall body growth; ACTH (adrenocorticotropic hormone), which controls steroid hormone secretion by the adrenal cortex; thyrotropic hormone, which stimulates the activity of the thyroid gland; and three gonadotropic hormones, which control growth and reproductive activity of the gonads (ovaries and testes). The posterior lobe secretes antidiuretic hormone, which causes water retention by the kidneys, and oxytocin, which stimulates the mammary glands to release milk and also causes uterine contractions. An overactive pituitary during childhood can cause gigantism; during adulthood, it can cause acromegaly. Dwarfism results from pituitary deficiency in childhood. See also Acromegaly.

**PLACEBO:**
An inactive substance against which investigational treatments are compared for efficacy. See also Placebo Controlled Study.

**PLACEBO CONTROLLED STUDY:**
A method of investigation of drugs in which an inactive substance (the placebo) is given to one group of patients, while the drug being tested is given to another group. The results obtained in the two groups are then compared.

**PLACEBO EFFECT:**
A physical or emotional change occurring after a substance is taken or administered that is not the result of any special property of the substance. The change may be beneficial, reflecting the expectations of the patient and, often, the expectations of the person giving the substance.

**PLASMA:**
That 10 percent of the blood that contains nutrients, electrolytes (dissolved salts), gases, albumin, clotting factors, wastes and hormones.

**PLASMA CELLS:**
Large antibody-producing cells that develop from B cells. See also Antibodies; B Lymphocytes.

**PLASMAPHERESIS:**
The selective removal of certain proteins or antibodies from the blood (followed by reinjection of the blood). This process is sometimes used in the treatment of some peripheral neuropathies and is an integral part of passive immunotherapies for HIV. See also Neuropathy.

**PLATELETS:**
Active agents of inflammation when damage occurs to a blood vessel. They are not actually cells, but fragments released by megakaryocyte cells. Megakaryocyte is a large cell in the bone marrow whose function is to produce platelets. When vascular damage (i.e., damage to blood

vessels) occurs, the platelets stick to the vascular walls, forming clots to prevent the loss of blood. Thus, it is important to have adequate numbers of normally functioning platelets to maintain effective coagulation of the blood. There are drugs that can potentially alter the platelet count, making it necessary to monitor the count. Also, some people with HIV infection develop thrombocytopenia (a condition characterized by a platelet count of less than 100,000 platelets per cubic millimeter of blood). The normal value for men is 154,000–354,000 platelets per cubic millimeter of blood. For women, it is 162,000–380,000 platelets per cubic millimeter of blood.

### PML:
See Progressive Multifocal Leukoencephalopathy.

### PNEUMOCYSTIS CARINII PNEUMONIA (PCP):
1. A protozoal infection of the lungs. 2. A life-threatening lung infection that can affect people with weakened immune systems, such as those infected with HIV. More than three-quarters of all people with HIV disease will develop PCP if they do not receive treatment to prevent it. The standard treatment for people with PCP is either a combination of trimethoprim and sulfamethoxazole (TMP/SMX, also called Bactrim or Septra) or pentamidine. See also Pentamidine; Protozoa.

### POLYMERASE:
Any of several enzymes that catalyze the formation of DNA or RNA from precursor substances in the presence of preexisting DNA or RNA acting as templates (i.e., patterns). See also DNA; Enzyme; Ribonucleic Acid.

### POLYMERASE CHAIN REACTION (PCR):
1. A laboratory process that selects a DNA segment from a mixture of DNA chains and rapidly replicates it; used to create a large, readily analyzed sample of a piece of DNA. It is used in DNA fingerprinting and in medical tests to identify diseases from the infectious agent's DNA. See also DNA. 2. As related to HIV: A sensitive laboratory

technique that can detect and quantify HIV in a person's blood or lymph node.

**POLYNEURITIS:**
Inflammation of many nerves at once.

**POLYVALENT VACCINE:**
A vaccine that is active against multiple viral strains.

**PRECURSOR CELLS:**
Cells from which other cells are formed by natural processes.

**PREVALENCE:**
A measure of the proportion of people in a population affected with a particular disease at a given time.

**PROCTITIS:**
Inflammation of the rectum.

**PRODROME:**
A symptom that indicates the onset of a disease.

**PROGENITOR:**
Parent or ancestor.

**PROGRESSIVE MULTIFOCAL LEUKOENCEPHALOPATHY (PML):**
An opportunistic infection resulting from reactivation or new infection with the JC virus. See also Opportunistic Infection.

**PROPHYLAXIS:**
Treatment that helps to prevent a disease or condition before it occurs or recurs.

**PROTEASE:**
An enzyme that hydrolyzes (i.e., breaks down) proteins to their component peptides. See also Enzyme; Peptide; Proteins.

**PROTEASE INHIBITORS:**
HIV protease is an aspartyl enzyme essential to the replicative life cycle of HIV. The three-dimensional molecular structure of the HIV protease has been fully determined. Pharmaceutical developers are therefore able to rationally design compounds to inhibit it and thus interfere with replication of the virus. In the US, five peptide-based protease inhibitors (saquinavir, Roche; A–80987, ABT–538, Abbott Laboratories; L735,524, Merck; KNI–272, NCI) are in clinical development. All compounds inhibit HIV-1 in vitro in nanomolar concentrations. In Europe, two peptide-based compounds (ABT–987, Abbott Laboratories; AG–1343, Agouron Pharmaceuticals, Inc.) are currently in development. See also In Vitro.

**PROTEINS:**
Any of the group of highly complex organic compounds found in all living cells. Protein is the most abundant class of all biological molecules, comprising about 50 percent of cellular dry weight. Classified by biological function, proteins include the enzymes, which catalyze cellular reactions; collagen, keratin and elastin, which are structural, or support, proteins; hemoglobin and other transport proteins; casein, ovalbumin and other nutrient proteins; antibodies, which are necessary for immunity; protein hormones, which regulate metabolism; and proteins such as actin and myosin, the contractile muscle proteins that perform mechanical work. Structurally, proteins are large molecules composed of one or more chains of varying amounts of the same 22 amino acids, which are linked by peptide bonds. Each protein is characterized by a unique and invariant amino acid sequence. Protein chains may contain hundreds of amino acids; some proteins also incorporate phosphorus or such metals as iron, zinc and copper. The amino acid sequence also determines the molecule's three-dimensional structure; this so-called native state is required for proper biological

function. The information for the syntheses of the specific amino acid sequences from free amino acids is carried by the cell's nucleic acid. See also Peptide; Ribonucleic Acid.

**PROTOCOL:**
The detailed plan for a clinical trial that states the trial's rationale, purpose, drug or vaccine dosages, length of study, routes of administration, who may participate and other aspects of trial design. See also Clinical Trial; Inclusion/Exclusion Criteria.

**PROTOPLASM:**
Fundamental material composing all living things. Protoplasm, which exists in all plants and animals in the small units called cells, is mainly (85–90 percent) water and also contains proteins, fatty substances and inorganic salts. It is always enclosed by a thin surface membrane that controls the passage of materials into and out of the cell. It displays the general properties associated with life—the capacity to respond to stimuli and the ability to perform the essential physiological functions.

**PROTOZOA:**
A group of one-celled animals. Some protozoa can cause human disease.

**PSEUDOVIRION:**
A virus-like particle.

**PUBLIC HEALTH SERVICE (PHS):**
A multi-agency organizational component of the US Department of Health and Human Services. See also Centers for Disease Control and Prevention; Health Resources and Services Administration; National Institutes of Health.

**PULMONARY:**
Pertaining to the lungs.

# R

**RANDOMIZED TRIAL:**
A study in which participants are randomly assigned to either a treatment arm or placebo arm of a clinical trial. See also Clinical Trial; Placebo.

**REACTOGENICITY:**
The capacity to produce adverse reactions.

**RECEPTOR:**
A molecule on the surface of a cell that serves as a recognition or binding site for antigens, antibodies or other cellular or immunological components. See also Antibodies; Antigen.

**RECOMBINANT:**
An organism whose genome contains integrated genetic material from a different organism. See also Genome.

**RECOMBINANT DNA:**
See Biotechnology; Genetic Engineering.

**REGULATORY GENES:**
As related to HIV: Three regulatory HIV genes—tat, rev and nef—and three so-called auxiliary genes—vif, vpr and vpu—contain information for the production of proteins that control (i.e., regulate) the virus's ability to infect a cell, produce new copies of the virus or cause disease. See also nef; rev; tat.

**REGULATORY T CELLS:**
T cells that direct other immune cells to perform special functions. The chief regulatory cell, the CD4+ T cell or T helper cell, is HIV's chief target. See also CD4 (T4) or CD4+ Cells; T Cells.

**REMISSIONS:**
The lessening of the severity or duration of outbreaks of a disease, or the abatement (diminution in degree or intensity) of symptoms altogether over a period of time.

**RENAL:**
Pertaining to the kidneys.

**RETICULOENDOTHELIAL CELLS:**
A system of interstitial cells that includes all the phagocytic cells, which trap and consume foreign agents, except the leukocytes circulating in the bloodstream. This system forms a network throughout the body and is another of the body's defense systems against invading organisms in the connective tissues of the body. See also Leukocytes; Phagocyte.

**RETINA:**
Light-sensitive tissue at the back of the eye that transmits visual impulses via the optic nerve to the brain.

**RETINITIS:**
Inflammation of the retina, linked in AIDS to CMV infection. Untreated, it can lead to blindness. See also Cytomegalovirus; Retina.

**RETROVIRUS:**
HIV and other viruses that carry their genetic material in the form of RNA and that have the enzyme reverse transcriptase. Like all viruses, HIV can replicate only inside cells, commandeering the cell's machinery to reproduce. Like other retroviruses, HIV uses the enzyme called reverse transcriptase to convert its RNA into DNA, which is then integrated into the host cell DNA. See also DNA; Reverse Transcriptase; Ribonucleic Acid.

## REV:

One of the regulatory genes of the HIV virus. Three HIV regulatory genes—tat, rev and nef—and three so-called auxiliary genes—vif, vpr and vpu—contain information necessary for the production of proteins that control the virus's ability to infect a cell, produce new copies of the virus or cause disease. See also nef; tat.

## REVERSE TRANSCRIPTASE:

This enzyme of the HIV virus (and other retroviruses) converts the single-stranded viral RNA into DNA, the form in which the cell carries its genes. The antiviral drugs approved in the US for the treatment of HIV infection—AZT, ddC and ddI—all work by interfering with this stage of the viral life cycle. See also AZT; ddC; ddI; DNA; Ribonucleic Acid.

## RIBONUCLEIC ACID (RNA):

1. A nucleic acid, found mostly in the cytoplasm of cells, that is important in the synthesis of proteins. The amount of RNA varies from cell to cell. RNA, like the structurally similar DNA, is a chain made up of subunits called nucleotides. In protein synthesis, messenger RNA (mRNA) replicates the DNA code for a protein and moves to sites in the cell called ribosomes. There, transfer RNA (tRNA) assembles amino acids to form the protein specified by the messenger RNA. Most forms of RNA (including messenger and transfer RNA) consist of a single nucleotide strand, but a few forms of viral RNA that function as carriers of genetic information (instead of DNA) are double-stranded. 2. A nucleic acid associated with the control of chemical activities inside a cell. One type of RNA transfers information from the cell's DNA to the protein-forming system of a cell outside the nucleus. Some viruses (e.g., HIV) carry RNA instead of the more usual genetic material DNA. See also Cytoplasm; DNA; Retrovirus.

## RIBOSOME:

A cytoplasmic organelle composed of ribonucleic acid and protein that functions in the synthesis of protein. Ribosomes interact with messenger RNA and transfer RNA to join together amino acid units into a polypeptide chain according to the sequence determined by the genetic code. See also Cytoplasm; Ribonucleic Acid.

### RNA:
See Ribonucleic Acid.

### ROUTE OF ADMINISTRATION:
See Administration.

### RYAN WHITE CARE ACT:
The Ryan White Comprehensive AIDS Resources Emergency (CARE) Act of 1990 represents the largest dollar investment made by Congress to date specifically for the provision of services for people with HIV infection. The purpose of the Act is "to improve the quality and availability of care for individuals and families with HIV disease."

# S

**SEBORRHEIC DERMATITIS:**
A chronic inflammatory disease of the skin of unknown etiology (i.e., cause or origin), characterized by moderate erythema; dry, moist or greasy scaling; and yellow crusted patches on various areas, including the mid-parts of the face, ears, supraorbital regions (above the orbit of the eye), umbilicus (the navel), genitalia, and especially the scalp. See also Erythematous.

**SEROCONVERSION:**
The development of antibodies to a particular antigen. When people develop antibodies to HIV or an experimental HIV vaccine, they "seroconvert" from antibody-negative to antibody-positive. See also Antibodies; Antigen.

**SEROLOGIC TEST:**
Any of a number of tests that are performed on the clear portion of blood (serum). Often refers to a test that determines the presence of antibodies to antigens such as viruses. See also Antibodies; Antigen; Serum.

**SEROPREVALENCE:**
As related to HIV infection: The proportion of persons who have serologic (i.e., pertaining to serum) evidence of HIV infection at any given time. See also Serum.

**SEROSTATUS:**
Results of a test for specific antibodies. See also Antibodies.

**SERUM:**
The clear, thin and sticky fluid portion of the blood that remains after coagulation. Serum contains no blood cells, platelets or fibrinogen.

### SEXUALLY TRANSMITTED DISEASE (STD):

Also called venereal disease. A contagious disease usually acquired by sexual intercourse or genital contact. Historically, the five venereal diseases were: gonorrhea, syphilis, chancroid, granuloma inguinale and lymphogranuloma venereum. To these have been added scabies, herpes genitalis and anorectal herpes and warts, pediculosis, trichomoniasis, genital candidiasis, molluscum contagiosum, nonspecific urethritis, chlamydial infections, cytomegalovirus and AIDS. See also Herpes Simplex Virus II; Molluscum Contagiosum.

### SF-2:

A strain of HIV used in vaccine development.

### SHINGLES:

See Herpes Varicella Zoster Virus.

### SHIV:

Genetically engineered hybrid virus having an HIV envelope and an SIV core. See also Genetic Engineering; Hybrid; Simian Immunodeficiency Virus.

### SIDE EFFECTS:

The action or effect of a drug (or vaccine) other than that desired. The term usually refers to undesired or negative effects, such as headache, skin irritation or liver damage. Experimental drugs must be evaluated for both immediate and long-term side effects.

### SIMIAN IMMUNODEFICIENCY VIRUS (SIV):

An HIV-like virus that infects monkeys, chimpanzees and other nonhuman primates.

### SIV:

See Simian Immunodeficiency Virus.

**SPINAL TAP:**
See Lumbar Puncture.

**SPLENOMEGALY:**
An enlarged spleen.

**STANDARDS OF CARE:**
Treatment regimen or medical management based on state-of-the-art patient care.

**STATISTICAL SIGNIFICANCE:**
A term based on statistical tests that is used to denote the probability that the observed association could have occurred by chance alone. Does not refer to medical or biological significance of an association. For example, a statistical significance at the 1-percent level indicates a 1-in-100 chance that a result can be ascribed to chance.

**STD:**
See Sexually Transmitted Disease.

**STEM CELLS:**
Cells from which all blood cells derive. Bone marrow is rich in stem cells.

**STERILIZING IMMUNITY:**
An immune response that completely eliminates an infection.

**STEVENS-JOHNSON SYNDROME:**
A severe and sometimes fatal form of erythema multiforme that is characterized by conjunctivitis (eye inflammation) and often results in blindness, Vincent's angina (trench mouth) and ulceration of the genitals and anus. See also Erythema Multiforme.

## STOMATITIS:

Any of numerous inflammatory diseases of the mouth having various causes, such as mechanical trauma, irritants, allergy, vitamin deficiency or infection.

## STRATIFICATION:

A layered configuration.

## SUBARACHNOID SPACE:

The space through which the spinal fluid circulates.

## SUBCLINICAL INFECTION:

An infection, or phase of infection, without readily apparent symptoms or signs of disease.

## SUBCUTANEOUS:

Beneath or introduced beneath the skin (e.g., subcutaneous injections).

## SUBUNIT HIV VACCINE:

A genetically engineered vaccine that is based on only part of the HIV molecule. See also Genetic Engineering.

## SULFA DRUG:

Any of a class of synthetic chemical substances derived from sulfanilamide and used to treat bacterial infections. These drugs inhibit the action of para-aminobenzoic acid, a substance bacteria needed in order to reproduce. Sulfa drugs are used primarily in the treatment of urinary tract infections and ulcerative colitis. Antibiotics have largely replaced them in the treatment of other bacterial infections.

## SULFONAMIDES:

See Sulfa Drug.

## SUPERANTIGEN:

Investigators have proposed that a molecule known as a superantigen, either made by HIV or an unrelated agent, may stimulate massive quantities of CD4+ T cells at once, rendering them highly susceptible to HIV infection and subsequent cell death. See also Antigen; CD4 (T4) or CD4+ Cells.

## SUPPRESSOR T CELLS:

(T8, CD8). Subset of T cells that halt antibody production and other immune responses. See also Antibodies; T Cells.

## SURROGATE MARKER:

A substitute; a person or thing that replaces another. In HIV disease, the number of CD4+ T cells and CD8+ cells is a surrogate immunological marker of disease progression. See also CD4 (T4) or CD4+ Cells; CD8 (T8) Cells.

## SURVEILLANCE:

Close or continuous observation or testing (e.g., serosurveillance), used, among others, in epidemiology. Immunological surveillance, or immunosurveillance, is a monitoring process of the immune system that detects and destroys neoplastic (e.g., cancerous) cells and that tends to break down in immunosuppressed individuals. See also Epidemiologic Surveillance.

## SUSCEPTIBLE:

Vulnerable or predisposed to a disease.

## SYMPTOMS:

Any perceptible, subjective change in the body or its functions that indicates disease or phases of disease, as reported by the patient.

## SYNCYTIA:

("Giant Cells"). Dysfunctional multicellular clumps formed by cell-to-cell fusion. Cells infected with HIV may also fuse with nearby uninfected cells, forming balloonlike giant cells called syncytia. In test tube experiments, these giant cells have been associated with the death of uninfected cells. The presence of so-called syncytia-inducing variants of HIV has been correlated with rapid disease progression in HIV-infected individuals.

**SYNDROME:**
A group of symptoms and diseases that together are characteristic of a specific condition.

**SYNERGISM/SYNERGISTIC:**
An interaction between two or more agents (drugs) that produces or enhances an effect that is greater than the sum of the effects produced by the individual agents.

**SYNTHESIS:**
1. In chemistry, the formation of a compound from simpler compounds or elements. 2. The production of a substance (e.g., as in protein synthesis) by the union of chemical elements, groups or simpler compounds, or by the degradation (i.e., breaking down) of a complex compound.

**SYPHILIS:**
A disease (usually sexually transmitted) resulting from infection with the spirochete (a bacterium) *Treponema pallidum*.

# T

## TAT:
One of the regulatory genes of the HIV virus. Three HIV regulatory genes—tat, rev and nef—and three so-called auxiliary genes—vif, vpr and vpu—contain information necessary for the production of proteins that control the virus's ability to infect a cell, produce new copies of the virus or cause disease. The tat gene is thought to enhance virus replication. See also nef; rev.

## TB:
See Tuberculosis.

## T CELLS:
(T Lymphocytes). A thymus-derived white blood cell that participates in a variety of cell-mediated immune reactions. Three fundamentally different types of T cells are recognized: helper, killer and suppressor (each has many subdivisions). T lymphocytes are CD3+ and can be separated into the CD4+ T helper cells and the CD8+ cytotoxic/suppresssor cells. See also Thymus.

## TEMPLATE:
A gauge, pattern or mold used as a guide to the form of the piece being made. In biology, a molecule (such as DNA) that serves as a pattern for the generation of another macromolecule (e.g., messenger RNA).

## TERATOGENICITY:
The production of physical defects in offspring in utero (i.e., causing birth defects).

## TERRY BEIRN COMMUNITY PROGRAMS FOR CLINICAL RESEARCH ON AIDS (CPCRA):

The National Institute of Allergy and Infectious Diseases (NIAID) started the CPCRA in 1989, adding Terry Beirn's name in 1991 in honor of the late, former manager of the American Foundation for AIDS Research and health policy consultant for Senator Edward Kennedy. CPCRA is one of four HIV clinical trials programs supported by NIAID. See also National Institute of Allergy and Infectious Diseases; Community Programs for Clinical Research on AIDS.

## THERAPEUTIC HIV VACCINE:

A vaccine designed to boost the immune response to HIV in persons already infected with the virus.

## 3TC:

Also known as Lamivudine, 3TC is composed of the (—) enantiomer of the racemic mixture 2′-deoxy-3′-thiacytidine. Like other nucleoside analogs, 3TC inhibits HIV replication through viral DNA chain termination. It has been used in clinical trials in combination with AZT. See also AZT; Nucleoside Analog.

## THROMBOCYTOPENIA:

A decreased number of blood platelets (cells important for blood clotting). See also Platelets.

## THRUSH:

Sore patches in the mouth caused by the fungus *Candida albicans*. Thrush is one of the most frequent early symptoms of an immune disorder. The fungus commonly lives in the mouth, but only causes problems when the body's resistance is reduced either by antibiotics that have reduced the number of competitive organisms in the mouth, or by an immune deficiency such as HIV disease. See also *Candida*.

## THYMOSIN:
A polypeptide hormone of the thymus that influences the maturation of T cells destined for an active role in cell-mediated immunity. See also T Cells; Thymus.

## THYMUS:
A mass of glandular tissue located in the neck or chest of most vertebrates. Found in the upper chest under the breastbone in humans, the thymus is essential to the development of the body's system of immunity beginning in fetal life (i.e., before birth). The thymus processes white blood cells, known as lymphocytes, which kill foreign cells and stimulate other immune cells to produce antibodies. The gland grows throughout childhood until puberty and then gradually decreases in size. See also Antibodies; Lymphocyte.

## TISSUE:
A collection of similar cells acting together to perform a particular function. There are four basic tissues in the body: epithelial, connective, muscle and nerve.

## TITER:
(Also "titre"). A laboratory measurement of the amount (or concentration) of a given compound in solution.

## T LYMPHOCYTE PROLIFERATION ASSAY:
Measures the strength of response of T memory cells (a subgroup of T lymphocytes) to HIV. See also T Cells.

## T LYMPHOCYTES:
See T Cells.

## TOXICITY:
The extent, quality or degree of being poisonous or harmful to the body.

## TOXOPLASMOSIS:

Toxoplasmosis is an infection that is caused by the protozoan parasite *Toxoplasma gondii*. The parasite is carried by cats, birds and other animals and is found in soil contaminated by cat feces and in meat, particularly pork. The parasite can infect the lungs, retina of the eye, heart, pancreas, liver, colon and testes. Once *T. gondii* invades the body, it remains there, but the immune system in a healthy person usually prevents the parasite from causing disease. If the immune system becomes severely damaged, as in people with AIDS, or is suppressed by drugs, *T. gondii* can begin to multiply and cause severe disease. The most common site of toxoplasmosis is the brain. When *T. gondii* invades the brain, causing inflammation, the condition is called toxoplasmic encephalitis. While the disease can occur in persons with healthy immune systems, it can normally be cured successfully. See also Protozoa.

## TRANSAMINASE:

A liver enzyme. A laboratory test that measures transaminase levels is used to assess the health of the liver.

## TRANSCRIPTION:

The process of constructing a messenger RNA molecule using a DNA molecule as a template with the resulting transfer of genetic information to the messenger RNA. As related to HIV: The process by which the provirus produces new viruses. RNA copies called messenger RNA must be made that can be read by the host cell's protein-making machinery. Transcription is facilitated by cellular enzymes, including RNA polymerase II. The viral genes may partly control this process: tat, for example, encodes a protein that accelerates the transcription process by binding to a section of the newly made viral RNA. See also Integration; Messenger RNA; tat; Template.

## TRANSFER FACTOR:

A fraction of white blood cells that apparently "transfers" capability to mount an immune response to a specific antigen. See also Antigen.

**TRANSFUSION:**
1. The process of transfusing fluid (such as blood) into a vein. 2. The transfer of whole blood or blood products from one individual to another.

**TRANSLATION:**
As related to HIV: The process by which HIV messenger RNA is processed in a cell's nucleus and transported to the cytoplasm, the cellular material outside the nucleus. In the cytoplasm, the cell's protein-making machinery translates the messenger RNA into viral protein and enzymes. See also Cytoplasm; Enzyme; Messenger RNA; Nucleus.

**TRANSMISSION:**
In the context of HIV disease: HIV is spread most commonly by sexual contact with an infected partner. The virus can enter the body through the mucosal lining of the vagina, vulva, penis, rectum or, very rarely, the mouth during sex. The likelihood of transmission is increased by factors that may damage these linings, especially other sexually transmitted diseases that cause ulcers or inflammation. Studies of SIV infection of the genital membranes of nonhuman primates suggest that the sentinel cells known as mucosal dendritic cells may be the first cells infected. Infected dendritic cells may migrate to lymph nodes and infect other cells. HIV also is spread through contact with infected blood, most often by the sharing of drug needles or syringes contaminated with minute quantities of blood containing the virus. Children can contract HIV from their infected mothers either during pregnancy or birth, or postnatally, via breastfeeding. Current research indicates that the AIDS virus may be 100 to 1000 times more contagious during the first two months of infection, when routine AIDS tests are unable to tell whether people are infected. See also Lymph Nodes; Simian Immunodeficiency Virus.

**TREATMENT IND:**
A program to provide experimental treatments to a class of patients who lack satisfactory alternative treatment. IND stands for Investigational New Drug application, which is part of the process to get approval from the Food and Drug Administration for marketing a new prescription drug in the US. See also Investigational New Drug.

**TUBERCULOSIS (TB):**
A bacterial infection caused by *Mycobacterium tuberculosis*. TB bacteria are spread by airborne droplets expelled from the lungs when a person with active TB coughs, sneezes or speaks. Repeated exposure to these droplets can lead to infection in the air sacs of the lungs. The immune defenses of healthy people usually prevent TB infection from spreading beyond a very small area of the lungs. If the body's immune system is impaired because of infection with HIV, aging, malnutrition or other factors, the TB bacterium may begin to spread more widely in the lungs or to other tissues.

# U

**UTERUS:**

A hollow muscular organ located in the pelvic cavity of female mammals in which the fertilized egg implants and develops. Also called womb.

### V3 LOOP:
Section of the gp120 protein on the surface of HIV. Appears to be important in stimulating neutralizing antibodies. See also Antibodies; gp120.

### VACCINATION:
Inoculation of a substance (vaccine) into the body for the purpose of producing active immunity against a disease. The vaccine is usually a weakened culture of the agent causing the disease; the use of vaccines is a cornerstone of preventive medicine. Vaccination was used in ancient times in China, India and Persia, and was introduced to the West in the late 18th century by E. Jenner. Vaccinations have eradicated smallpox and are used today to prevent diphtheria, poliomyelitis, rabies and typhoid. Experimental vaccines for certain cancers have been developed for laboratory mice. See also Inoculation.

### VACCINE:
A substance that contains antigenic components from an infectious organism. By stimulating an immune response (but not disease), it protects against subsequent infection by that organism. See also Antigen; Vaccination.

### VACCINIA:
A cowpox virus, formerly used in human smallpox vaccines. Employed as a vector in HIV vaccine research to transport HIV genes into the body. See also Vaccination; Vector.

### VARIABLE REGION:
The part of an antibody's structure that differs from one antibody to another. See also Antibodies.

## VECTOR:

A nonpathogenic bacterium or virus used to transport an antigen into the body to stimulate protective immunity (e.g., in a vaccine). See also Antigen.

## VIRAL BURDEN:

(Viral Load). The amount of HIV virus in the circulating blood. Monitoring a person's viral burden is important because of the apparent correlation between the amount of virus in the blood and the severity of the disease: sicker patients generally have more virus than those with less advanced disease. A new, sensitive, rapid test—called the branched DNA assay for HIV-1 infection—can be used to monitor the HIV viral burden. In the future, this procedure may help clinicians to decide when to give anti-HIV therapy. It may also help investigators determine more quickly if experimental HIV therapies are effective.

## VIRAL CORE:

1. Typically a virus contains an RNA (ribonucleic acid) or DNA (deoxyribonucleic acid) core of genetic material surrounded by a protein coat. See also DNA; Ribonucleic Acid. 2. As related to HIV: Within HIV's envelope is a bullet-shaped core made of another protein, p24, that surrounds the viral RNA. Each strand of HIV RNA contains the virus's nine genes. Three of these—gag, pol and env—are structural genes that contain information needed to make structural proteins. The env gene, for example, codes for gp160, a protein that is later broken down to gp120 and gp41. See also env; gp41; gp120; gp160; p24.

## VIRAL CULTURE:

A laboratory method for growing viruses.

## VIRAL ENVELOPE:

As related to HIV: HIV is spherical in shape with a diameter of 1/10,000 of a millimeter. The outer coat, or envelope, is composed of two layers of fat-like molecules called lipids, taken from the membranes of human cells. Embedded in the envelope are numerous cellular proteins, as well as mushroom-shaped HIV proteins that protrude from the surface. Each mushroom is thought to consist of a cap made of four glycoprotein molecules called gp120, and a stem consisting of four gp41 molecules embedded in the envelope. The virus uses these proteins to attach to and infect cells.

**VIRAL LOAD:**
See Viral Burden.

**VIREMIA:**
The presence of virus in the bloodstream.

**VIRION:**
A virus particle existing freely outside a host cell. A mature virus.

**VIROLOGY:**
The study of viruses and viral disease.

**VIRUCIDE:**
Any agent that destroys or inactivates a virus.

**VIRUS:**
Organism composed mainly of nucleic acid within a protein coat, ranging in size from 100 to 2000 angstroms (unit of length; 1 angstrom is equal to $10^{-10}$ meters); they can be seen only with an electron microscope. During the stage of their life cycle when they are free and infectious, viruses do not carry out the usual functions of living cells, such as respiration and growth; however, when they enter a living plant, animal or bacterial cell, they make use of the host cell's chemical energy and protein– and nucleic acid–synthesizing ability to replicate themselves. Viral nucleic acids are single— or double-stranded and may be DNA (deoxyribonucleic acid) or RNA (ribonucleic acid). After viral components are made by the infected host cell, virus particles are released; the host cell is often dissolved. Some viruses do not kill cells but transform them into a cancerous state; some cause illness and then

seem to disappear, while remaining latent and later causing another, sometimes much more severe, form of disease. Viruses, known to cause cancer in animals, are suspected of causing cancer in humans. Viruses also cause measles, mumps, yellow fever, poliomyelitis, influenza and the common cold. Some viral infections can be treated with drugs. See also DNA; Nucleic Acid; Ribonucleic Acid.

**VISCERAL:**
Pertaining to the major internal organs.

# W

**WASTING SYNDROME:**
The HIV wasting syndrome involves involuntary weight loss of 10 percent of baseline body weight plus either chronic diarrhea (two loose stools per day for more than 30 days) or chronic weakness and documented fever (for 30 days or more, intermittent or constant) in the absence of a concurrent illness or condition other than HIV infection that would explain the findings.

**WESTERN BLOT:**
A laboratory test for the presence of specific antibodies, more accurate than the ELISA test. See also Antibodies; ELISA.

# SOURCES

**AIDS Clinical Care**, Vol. 7, No. 1 (January 1995). A.R. Rabson, Enumeration of T-Cell Subsets in Patients with HIV Infection, pp. 1–3.

**AIDS/HIV Treatment Directory**. American Foundation for AIDS Research. Vol. 2, No. 2 (August 1988); Vol. 7, No. 4 (January 1995).

**AIDS Mood Upbeat—For a Change**, by John Cohen. *Science*, Vol. 267, No. 5200 (February 17, 1995), pp. 959–960.

**American Heritage Dictionary of the English Language, Third Edition**. New York: Houghton Mifflin, 1992.

**CDC National Serosurveillance Summary, Vol. 3**. Atlanta: Centers for Disease Control and Prevention, 1992.

**Clinical Manual for Care of the Adult Patient With HIV Infection**. Edited by H. Libmen, M.D., and R.A. Witzburg, M.D. Boston: Boston City Hospital, Department of Medicine, 1990.

**Concise Columbia Encyclopedia**. New York: Columbia University Press, 1991.

**Dendritic Cells: A Key to Early HIV Infection**. NIAID News. Rockville, Maryland: National Institute of Allergy and Infectious Diseases, January 30, 1995.

**Dorland's Illustrated Medical Dictionary, 28th Edition**. Philadelphia: W.B. Saunders Company, 1988.

**Emerging Fungal Threat**, by S. Sterber. *Science*, Vol. 266, No. 5191 (December 9, 1994), pp. 1632–1634.

**Exposure to Hepatatis C Virus Does Not Protect Against Reinfections, Dimming Hopes for a Protective Vaccine**. NIAID Fact Sheet Update. Rockville, Maryland: National Institute of Allergy and Infectious Diseases, October 1, 1992.

**Fauci: Host Factors Key to Control of HIV Infection**. NIAID News. Rockville, Maryland: National Institute of Allergy and Infectious Diseases, January 30, 1995.

**Hepatitis**. NIAID Fact Sheet. Rockville, Maryland: National Institute of Allergy and Infectious Diseases, August 1992.

**HIV/AIDS and Opportunistic Infections**. NIAID Fact Sheet. Rockville, Maryland: National Institute of Allergy and Infectious Diseases, November 1994.

**HIV Vaccine Glossary**. Rockville, Maryland: National Institute of Allergy and Infectious Diseases, June 1994.

**How HIV Causes AIDS**. NIAID Backgrounder. Rockville, Maryland: National Institute of Allergy and Infectious Diseases, April 1994.

**Information Services for HIV/AIDS: Recommendations to the National Institutes of Health**. Report of a conference cosponsored by the National Library of Medicine and the NIH Office of AIDS Research, June 28–30, 1993. NIH Publication No. 94–3730 (January 1994).

**Interleukin-2 Produces Significant, Sustained Increase in CD4+ Cells in HIV-Infected People**. NIAID News. Rockville, Maryland: National Institute of Allergy and Infectious Diseases, March 1, 1995.

**Journal of Acquired Immunodeficiency Syndrome**, Vol. 3, No. 9 (1990): 896–903. Feingold, Anat R. et al. Cervical Cytologic Abnormalities and Papilloma Virus in Women Infected With Human Immunodeficiency Virus, September 1990.

**Mosby's Medical, Nursing, and Allied Health Dictionary, Fourth Edition**. Philadelphia: F.A. Davis, 1994.

**National AIDS Clearinghouse HIV Glossary**. Prepared by the CDC National AIDS Clearinghouse, Rockville, Maryland.

**National HIV Serosurveillance Summary, Vol 3, Results Through 1992**. Atlanta: Centers for Disease Control and Prevention, 1992.

**NIAID Interleukin-2 Study**. NIAID Fact Sheet. Rockville, Maryland: National Institute of Allergy and Infectious Diseases, March 1995.

**NIAID Researchers Report New Data on Non-Progressive HIV Infection**. NIAID News. Rockville, Maryland: National Institute of Allergy and Infectious Diseases, January 25, 1995.

**1993 Revised Classification System for HIV Infection and Expanded Surveillance Case Definition for AIDS Among Adolescents Through Adults**. *Morbidity and Mortality Weekly Report*, Vol. 41, No. RR–17. Available from the Centers for Disease Control and Prevention, Atlanta, Georgia.

**PID: Guidelines for Prevention, Detection and Management**. *Clinical Courier*, Vol. 10, No. 1 (January 1992). Available from the National Institute of Allergy and Infectious Diseases, Rockville, Maryland.

**Ryan White Comprehensive AIDS Resources Emergency (CARE) Act**. Resources and Services Database Style Sheet, July 21, 1992.

**Tabor Cyclopedic Medical Dictionary, 15th Edition**. Edited by C.L. Thomas. Philadelphia: F.A. Davis Company, 1987.

**Test for HIV Viral Burden Promising in Clinical Setting**. NIAID News. Rockville, Maryland: National Institute of Allergy and Infectious Diseases, October 26, 1994.

**Webster's Encyclopedic Unabridged Dictionary of the English Language**. Avenel, New Jersey: Gramercy Books, 1989.

**Webster's Medical Desk Dictionary**. Springfield, Massachusetts: Merriam—Webster, Inc., 1986.